■ The Financial Manager's Guide to

Managed Care & Integrated Delivery Systems

Strategies for Contracting, Compensation & Reimbursement

Paul R. DeMuro

IRWIN
Professional Publishing®
Chicago • London • Singapore

ISBN 1-55738-623-4

Printed in the United States of America

BB

   2 3 4 5 6 7 8 9 0

CB/BJS

To my father,
who during his life instilled in me
the drive to succeed,
the desire to be the best in my chosen field,
a love of life,
and a commitment to . . . *enjoy!*

To my wife, Susan
and my daughter, Melissa

Table of Contents

TABLE OF CONTENTS

Preface and Acknowledgments

I authored the *Financial Manager's Guide to Managed Care and Integrated Delivery Systems* not only for financial managers in the healthcare industry, but for anyone with an interest in our healthcare system. Although the book's subject matter is broad in that it discusses the evolution of indemnity healthcare insurance to managed care and integrated delivery systems (IDS), its succinct treatment of these subjects makes it an indispensable guide to the alphabet soup of managed care and IDS and to the specifics of capitation and IDS models.

Although other books may describe the types of managed care organizations and providers, the forms of provider payment, and managed care contracting, I do so in one easily readable text which tells the financial manager what he needs to know. I also discuss capitation as a preferred payment mechanism, and the need to align financial incentives, drawing on the practical information which I have developed over many years of practicing in the California managed care environment.

I discuss how the primary care physician is the gatekeeper within managed care systems, why specialists should be capitated and the steps for doing so. My practical approach to managed care also discusses the importance of the managed care relationship, who receives payment and who can accept risk.

For over a decade I have been involved in medical group development, physician hospital organizations (PHOs), management services organizations (MSOs), and fully integrated delivery systems. This experience has made it possible for me to highlight the important aspects of independent practice associations (IPAs), clinics or group practices without walls, PHOs, MSOs, medical foundations and integrated delivery systems in an understandable manner. I not only provide models of many forms of these entities, but also discuss many of their positive and negative features. My extensive experience in working with such models throughout the country provides an invaluable perspective.

I also discuss many of the difficult issues that are not typically addressed in a work of this kind, including physician payment mechanisms, the concept of managing care, and physician credentialing. In seeking to cover the full range of managed care and IDS issues, I discuss the interests and position of specialty medical groups, networks, and ancillary providers and what alternatives they present to fully integrated delivery systems.

I address the special position and challenges of academic medical centers, and I include a special chapter on alliance, contract or virtual integration where physicians link with a managed care plan to create a delivery system without the high cost of hospital services. A new idea I have addressed is the replication of the physician equity model. When it cannot be employed because of lack of physician capital, I pose alternatives to replicate that model. Finally, I highlight the major legal issues faced in managed care and IDS development and operations.

This book is an invaluable and unique work because in authoring it, I was able to draw upon my educational background as a CPA and an attorney with an MBA in finance, my professional experience working in managed care for over a decade, and working in the area of integrated delivery systems from a California perspective. My experience as a leading national legal architect in integrated delivery system development has made it possible for me to place these issues in a most interesting perspective.

This work would not have been possible without the support of my partners at Latham & Watkins, who have created a most special environment for the practice of law and creativity; my secretary, Louise Will, and my word processor Thomas MacEntee, who have spent countless hours working on this manuscript; Dick Clarke, the President of the Healthcare Financial Management Association (HFMA) and Doc Barto, who helped encourage me to author this work for the benefit of HFMA, its members, and those individuals interested in our healthcare system; and to my colleagues on HFMA's National Principles and Practices Board, who have for more than 20 years helped perfect the field of healthcare finance. A special thanks is due to my long-time mentor and friend, Len Homer, who introduced me to the field of healthcare in the late 1970s; and to my former partner, Russ Carpenter, who helped direct me into the area of managed care in 1982, and who pioneered integrated delivery systems soon thereafter. Finally, I could never have completed this book without the support of my wife, Susan, and my daughter, Melissa. Their understanding and sacrifice over the many months of late hours and weekend work this past year has been most special to me.

Paul R. DeMuro
Latham & Watkins
San Francisco and
Los Angeles, California

1

Background

In the early 1970s, those individuals in the United States who had healthcare coverage, and were not covered by Medicare or Medicaid, typically had healthcare coverage through their employers. The health benefits generally also covered their dependents. Occasionally, the employee had to pay a portion of the healthcare premium for his or her dependents, but often the employer paid all the premiums.

The nature of the healthcare benefits was indemnity insurance coverage. That is, the insurance company would indemnify the patient for a portion of the healthcare charges which the patient incurred for hospital or physician services. Typically, the patient assigned his or her benefits to the hospital and physician, thus permitting the insurance company to pay the hospital and physician directly.

Most indemnity plans had deductible amounts and coinsurance or copayments which would have to be paid by the patient. The deductible amount was the total of annual charges for hospital and physician services which the patient would have to pay prior to the insurance company paying any healthcare benefits. The coinsurance or copayment amount was the amount the patient would pay when the insurance company started to pay insurance benefits, after the deductible was reached. Typically this copayment would be 20% of the hospital and physician bills after the deductible amount, but subject to a cap. At some annual level, $5,000, $10,000, or more, the patient's responsibility to contribute 20% would cease, and the insurance company would pay 100% of the charges up to an annual limit of coverage. Beyond that limit, a major medical plan might also participate at 100% of the hospital and physician charges. Initially, many major medical plans did not have a cap on total healthcare benefits payable under the policy, although now many limit such benefits to $500,000 or $1,000,000 for the lifetime of the policy.

Although many health maintenance organizations (HMOs) existed—organizations which assume both the risk of financing and delivering physician and hospital services to an enrolled population for a fixed sum of money on a prepaid basis—their penetration was minimal except in certain areas where health plans such as Group Health Cooperative of Puget Sound in Washington and Kaiser Permanente Health Plan in California had a significant market share. Such health plans typically were closed systems where most of the physicians and hospitals participating in the system only provided services to the health plan beneficiaries. Many subsequent health plans have more open systems where the physicians and hospitals provide services to patients in addition to those of the contracting HMO.

As HMOs began to proliferate, they contracted with myriad hospitals and physicians in their attempt to create provider networks. Outside the closed-system HMOs, payments often were made to the physicians on a fee-schedule or other modified fee-for-service basis, and the hospitals were paid at charges or a discount from charges. The HMOs sought to control their costs principally through controls on utilization.

The Medicare program was introduced in the mid-1960s. No one could have imagined that the costs associated with the program would increase as rapidly as they did. Initially, hospitals were paid by Medicare on a cost-based reimbursement system. That is, payments to hospitals were based on the amount of costs or expenses which they incurred. As a result, the more costs incurred by a hospital through expansion and additional spending, the more costs passed through to Medicare. Although minimal limitations initially were placed on the reimbursability of costs by the Medicare program, the government increasingly placed further limitations on the reimbursement of such costs in the 1970s and thereafter.

Physicians were paid based on the lower of their usual and customary charges for a particular procedure, their actual charge for the procedure performed, or the prevailing physician charge in the community for services rendered to and procedures performed on Medicare patients. As a result, as charges increased, the cost to Medicare increased over time. The Medicare program sought to limit payments to physicians by limiting the prevailing charge in the community to an adjusted prevailing charge. Such a charge generally was one which was limited based on an index, and the limitation was set by a certain percentage increase to the charge which was allowable.

When the federal government began funding the state Medicaid programs, the states developed Medicaid plans which were approved by the federal government, and funded partly by the state and partly by the federal government. Many of these plans enacted reimbursement schemes similar to Medicare, where hospitals were paid on a cost basis and physicians were paid on a charge basis. Some states developed fee schedules for physician payments which either set or limited the payments to physicians. Some states implemented a rate setting policy for hospital payments, where a commission would determine the rates which hospitals could charge.

Many county hospitals sought to treat the poor and indigent who were not otherwise covered by Medicare or commercial health insurance. These facilities were supported primarily through federal, state, and county monies. With the addition of the Medicaid program, many of the patients treated by county hospitals were covered by that program. Often the county hospitals operated areawide trauma centers and complex emergency departments which were, in many instances, the only access that certain individuals had to physicians and medical care.

Inasmuch as hospital and physician charges were substantially lower than they are now, a number of individuals without insurance were able to pay all or part of their hospital and physician bills, however, even if over time. When unable to pay their bills, these self-pay patients became bad debts. Over time, the number of self-pay patients whose accounts became bad debts increased substantially.

As healthcare costs increased through the 1970s and early 1980s, there was much concern over how to stem the ever-rising rate of increase. Federal and state governments were increasingly concerned because of the strain on their budgets. The Medicare program, suffering from the burden of a cost-based system where costs to the program increased substantially each year, enacted the Medicare Prospective Payment System (PPS). Under this system, which was phased in through the middle 1980s, Medicare paid most hospitals a fixed amount per diagnosis related group (DRG), or disease, regardless of a patient's length of stay; although, for certain patients whose costs or length of stay might have been extraordinary and beyond a particular threshold, a hospital might be paid a cost- or day-outlier payment.

Capital costs were paid separately under a cost-based system until the enactment of the Medicare PPS system for capital cost payments in the early 1990s. Rehabilitation, long-term care, psychiatric care, and certain other facilities were not subject to the DRG payment system, but remained on a cost-based payment system. It was considered too difficult to convert these hospitals to a DRG system because of the nature of their patient population. In any event, the vast majority of all inpatient hospital Medicare payments would be payable to hospitals subject to DRG payments.

Hospitals soon had to learn how to manage the care for their Medicare inpatients in a more cost-effective manner because they would likely receive the same payment for a particular patient's illness even if they used excessive resources or if a patient stayed in the hospital a longer period of time. This management of care involved the judicious use of resources for which the hospital was financially responsible, and the management of a patient's stay in the hospital to ensure that its length was minimized.

Hospitals began to affiliate with, acquire, and make greater use of home health agencies in their discharge planning activities. Home health agencies provided skilled nursing services to patients in their homes, making it possible to discharge them earlier. Thus, if a Medicare patient could be sent home from the hospital a day or two earlier if the nursing services of a home health agency were available, the cost to the hospital of managing a patient's care would be less. In addition, Medicare would pay separately for covered home health agency services. Home health agency services were paid on a cost basis, subject to certain cost-of-visit limitations, and were not subject to payment under the DRG system. Thus, a hospital which properly employed the resources of a home health agency could discharge a patient earlier, realizing more margin on the inpatient stay; and, if the hospital owned a home health agency, begin receiving payment earlier for home health services, if the patient was discharged earlier.

Physicians, of course, have managed patient care or a patient's plan of treatment for years. Many, however, did not have the occasion to manage the cost of that care. In fact, with the implementation of the Medicare PPS, there were misaligned incentives for the hospitals and the physicians. As a hospital sought to decrease a Medicare patient's length of stay in the hospital, the physician treating the patient would have fewer opportunities to bill the Medicare program for encounters with the patient in the hospital. This misalignment of incentives, which also existed with respect to other payors, increased stress on the relationship between hospitals and physicians.

Many state Medicaid plans also sought to control costs in a number of ways. For example, California enacted Medi-Cal contracting, whereby, in certain areas, only those hospitals which reached agreement with the Medi-Cal program for contracts to provide inpatient hospital services to Medi-Cal beneficiaries were paid for nonemergency care to Medicaid inpatients. The hospitals were generally paid on a *per diem* basis (a set amount per day) for each hospitalized Medi-Cal patient. New Jersey enacted a form of DRG system, and Maryland was a rate-setting state, where a commission set hospital payment rates. Often, physician fees were limited by physician fee schedules, but hospital and physician incentives to manage care were rarely aligned.

In the early 1980s, preferred provider organizations (PPOs) began to emerge. These entities sought to contract with hospitals and physicians on a reduced fee-for-service basis with explicit or implicit promises of additional volume for these discounts. The hospitals and physicians who executed contracts with the PPO were known as preferred or participating providers. Many hospitals and physicians entered into such arrangements because they were fearful that if they did not do so, they would lose part of their existing patient base. In fact, many providers who entered into such contracts did retain much of their existing business, but at lower reimbursement rates and at reduced lengths of stay. Those that did not enter into such contracts occasionally found that their business declined.

Patients were supposed to be incentivized to visit preferred providers because if they did so, their deductible and copayment might be less. For example, a patient who visited a participating provider might have a $250 deductible and a 10% copayment, whereas a patient who visited a nonpreferred provider might have a $500 deductible and a 30% copayment. Obviously, the most popular PPOs were those that included a large number of providers, and more particularly those which included the provider the patient would have wanted to visit in any event. Thus, if a patient's personal physician was a participating provider, a patient might be more than satisfied with the arrangement because the patient's copayment would be reduced. The PPO would be satisfied if it contracted with the physicians for a discount which reduced its cost of physician services. The physician, however, would have merely offered a discount to retain the patient (or, as the physicians would soon realize, to retain the PPO's patient).

A form of PPO called an exclusive provider organization (EPO) also emerged. In this model, patients were required to obtain almost all their care through the providers which made up the exclusive provider network. Unless the EPO had a very large provider network, its ability to compete with this product initially was hindered by its exclusivity. However, it is easier to contain costs with an EPO because the EPO generally does not pay for many services outside of its network. An EPO may look somewhat like an HMO to the patient because the patient generally only visits EPO providers.

As healthcare costs continued to increase, PPOs and HMOs began to gain a greater share of the market because their cost to employers was less than indemnity policies. Hospitals discounted their rates to PPOs and HMOs, and physicians accepted fee schedules and offered discounts to these entities. Not all providers chose to participate in these arrangements with PPOs and HMOs, however, apparently hoping this move to such entities would be a short-lived fad. Over time, however, they began to realize that managed care was not a fad, and many providers who shunned certain contractual arrangements with health plans found it difficult to obtain such arrangements later. In fact, those providers who claimed that PPOs and HMOs were not for them because of quality of care concerns later found that, as the years passed, many PPOs and HMOs had enacted rigid credentialing and quality assurance programs, and were still paying at rates which the physicians believed were too low. The health plans, however, were seeking quality physicians. Some even required that most physicians be board certified. Thus, over time, it became clear that PPOs and HMOs were seeking both price and quality.

Many employer groups, health insurers, and PPOs soon realized what HMOs had known for years—that merely obtaining discounts from the providers in a system does not result in sufficiently containing the costs of providing healthcare services. HMOs, typically, require prior authorizations for admission of patients to hospitals, conduct continued stay and retrospective reviews, and manage the patient's plan of treatment. Unless an admission to a hospital was an emergency, the attending physician or hospital would have to telephone the health plan to receive prior authorization to admit the patient to the hospital. If the reasons for the admission met the requirements of the health plan, the patient could be admitted, and if the services were covered by the health plan, the health plan would generally pay for these services. The health plan, however, could deny payment for the admission on grounds that it was not medically necessary or the services to be rendered were noncovered services. In addition, if no prior authorization was sought, the plan might deny the admission retroactively solely on that basis and refuse payment.

Continued stay review is a review of a patient's care and treatment plan by the health plan when the patient is in the hospital. The health plan wants to ensure that the patient's treatment is progressing and that the patient is discharged from the hospital at the earliest possible date. The health plan reviewer, who is likely to be a nurse or other healthcare professional, might review the medical record and discuss the patient's care with his physician. Occasionally, a health plan might determine that no additional days in the hospital will be authorized for payment by the health plan. If the patient (or the patient in conjunction with his physician) elects to stay in the hospital, the patient might either request a reconsideration of the decision by the health plan or elect to pay for the remainder of the stay personally. A continued stay which is for the benefit of a patient's personal situation and is not medically necessary likely would be denied by a health plan. Whether the patient might be personally liable for the remainder of the stay, however, might depend upon whether the hospital provided such notice to the patient in writing and whether the patient signed an agreement or acknowledgment of such notice.

Most health plans occasionally conduct retrospective reviews of a patient's course of treatment at a hospital. Initially, such reviews were conducted to discuss with physicians their practice problems and to ensure more cost-effective and quality means of providing care for the future. However, many plans soon began to use such retrospective review mechanisms as a means to deny payment for care which they viewed as medically unnecessary, could have been provided in another setting, or for other reasons. Retrospective reviews, however, should not be as necessary if there have been continued stay reviews.

Initially, PPOs merely sought discounts from the ever-increasing charges for healthcare services which they experienced with providers. PPOs, however, soon began to develop characteristics which were similar to those of HMOs, particularly in the management of healthcare services. For example, PPOs began to require prior authorization for admission and treatment, continued stay, and retrospective review. Many even sought to closely manage the care of their patients, either on their own or through agents such as professional review organizations. These entities might seek to recommend to the health plan denials of payment for all or part of a patient's stay. Obviously, such an approach troubled providers who were now dealing with a third party, and for denials which were not current with a patient's stay (retroactive denials), in part because the professional review organization was not present to assess the patient's situation. It had to rely on medical records, notes in the records, and possible discussions with the patient's attending physician.

In the middle to late 1980s, as a result of the transition through the Medicare Prospective Payment System, technological advances, better utilization review, and management of care, the lengths of stay for patients at hospitals decreased dramatically. For example, a woman who delivered a baby by caesarian section once might have stayed in a hospital for seven days; now she stayed two or three. A patient who previously had surgery for kidney stones once might have stayed in the hospital a few weeks; now, instead of surgery, he might be treated with extracorporeal shock wave lithotripsy and be out in a day, or be treated as an outpatient.

At about the same time that lengths of stay began to drop, many of the hospitals' building projects began to come on line. In the mid-1980s, hospitals often sought to substantially expand their facilities because of demographic projections based upon utilization trends which suggested that additional hospital beds would be needed. Thus, hospitals were committed to building projects which were not, after all, as necessary as they once thought they were. Lengths of stay were decreasing, but additional hospital beds were coming on line.

Many of these commitments were exacerbated by the Certificate of Need (CON) process which existed in many states. Hospitals might have had to obtain the approval of a state agency to expand or construct existing facilities or add new hospital beds. Hospitals fearful that their competitors might be granted such approval wanted to ensure that their building projects were in the queue. As a result, they vigorously pursued CONs for more beds. By the time these approved projects were constructed in the late 1980s, many were not needed.

Many hospitals which had experienced an 85% occupancy in the mid-1980s saw occupancy drop to 40 to 60%, particularly with the addition of new space. As a result, the cost-per-patient stay and per day increased precipitously because the fixed costs for the hospitals had increased, and they were being spread over a smaller number of inpatients and days. While this phenomenon was taking place, health plans were seeking to reduce the increase in their rates of payments or rates of increase in their payments to providers.

As costs continued to increase, more HMOs sought to pay for the medical services to be received by their enrollees by capitating physicians—paying them a fixed amount per member per month (pmpm) for all physician and ancillary services which they might render to the enrollees for which they were financially responsible. Thus, the HMOs sought to shift substantial portions of the risk of treating their patient population to other parties. The physicians might only be capitated for the services they could provide, or they also might be capitated for additional services which they could not provide directly. Such services might include certain specialty physician and ancillary services.

As more and more physician groups began to receive capitated payments from HMOs for their physician services, physician groups began to design their own systems for prior authorization, review of care, and management through their networks. If the HMO was only providing the physicians with a fixed payment per member per month, the prior authorization, continued stay, and utilization review concerns of the plan were not as significant, and the physicians could adopt their own mechanisms. However, health plans wanted to be assured that the physician groups to whom they were paying capitation payments, and who were assuming certain functions of the health plans, would remain financially viable and were capable of employing systems which would result in the physician group operating in a cost-effective manner, while still providing quality care.

The primary care physician was seen as the focus for such managed care contracting because he or she acted as the gatekeeper. That is, the patient or enrollee's first encounter was with the primary care physician, the individual who authorized further treatment for the patient or made the referral to a subspecialist or specialist. As most healthcare resources are used or ordered by subspecialists and specialists, it became increasingly important for the primary care physician acting as the gatekeeper to refer to those specialists who were part of the network and practiced in a cost-effective manner. Typically, the specialists were paid on a modified fee-for-service basis, with the understanding that unless they received prior approval for certain procedures, they would not be paid for them. A shift later occurred to pay such specialists on a capitated basis to further control utilization.

It also was important for physicians who received payments under capitated contracts to ensure that they had arranged contracts with ancillary providers and suppliers for services, supplies, laboratory tests, or pharmaceuticals, for which the physicians were responsible. If the physicians assumed such financial risk, they had to negotiate contracts with such ancillary providers and suppliers for services which provided favorable rates to the physicians to maximize the value of the capitation payment to the physicians. Capitated arrangements with such providers and suppliers would reduce the physicians' risk, but often there were insufficient enrollees for the ancillary provider or supplier to agree to accept capitation. For example, a clinical laboratory might not agree to provide all necessary laboratory services for a patient population of only 1,000 lives. As a result, the physicians would have to negotiate a discount from charges or a fee schedule with the laboratory and control utilization.

As markets began to mature, it became increasingly evident to the physician providers that to the extent that they could subcapitate any providers or suppliers of ancillary services which they could not provide, they could substantially reduce their risk. When the number of lives which a physician group had under capitation increased, many ancillary providers and suppliers welcomed the opportunity to be capitated, as long as they could ensure that utilization would be controlled and they would not merely be doing the same tests or providing the same services as before, but at a substantially reduced rate.

On the physician side, the introduction by Medicare of the Resource Based Relative Value Scale (RBRVS) in 1992, which sought to realign payments to physicians under the Medicare program by decreasing certain payments to specialty physicians and increasing payments to primary care physicians, had the effect of reducing much physician reimbursement. The idea was to compensate better physicians' cognitive skills, and to realign or reduce the compensation to certain specialty physicians who were thought not to use as much time as may have been necessary in the past, in the provision of certain specialty services, and/or bring the payment of specialists more in line with the primary care physicians.

Many hospitals began to realize that being paid by the health plan on a modified fee-for-service or discount basis when a facility is being paid for a decreasing number of days might only exacerbate a hospital's financial problem. As a result, some hospitals, recognizing the positive effect which capitation had had on numerous physician groups, sought to negotiate with health plans for capitation payments. Their desire was in part based upon a recognition that hospitals in the evolving system were becoming cost centers, and that what was important was the ability to maintain a constant revenue stream and be a player in the healthcare system.

Hospitals which had previously been at the focal point of health systems because the more hospital services that were used, the more the hospital was paid, began to realize that if payments were limited, *e.g.*, through capitation, the hospitals were a cost to a system, not a revenue source. In fact, some providers even sought to obtain a percentage of the premium in lieu of capitation, believing that they could in fact partner with HMOs. Some HMOs, however, recognizing that much of their profit was generated by paying hospitals on a modified fee-for-service basis with strict utilization controls and from the risk pools shared with physicians because of decreased hospital utilization, were reluctant to capitate hospitals. That is, when physicians kept hospital utilization down, often the health plan would have money left over from what it budgeted for hospital care, which it would share with the physicians. Thus, physicians willing to accept capitation payments earlier in the decade made it more difficult, in some instances, for hospitals to convince health plans to capitate hospitals.

Specialty physicians, who generally were highly compensated in comparison to primary care physicians and who were previously seen by hospitals as the most important type of physician under a non-capitated system because their performance of procedures at the hospital brought it substantial revenues, soon became secondary in importance to primary care physicians. Under capitated managed care, the primary care physician is the gatekeeper and generally controls the revenue flow; as a result, the focus has shifted to the primary care physician.

In the early 1990s, integrated delivery systems (IDS)—which consist of at least the hospital and physician component for the provision of hospital and physician services, and possibly a managed care component—began to develop and proliferate. These systems sought to contract with managed care plans on behalf of both hospitals and physicians. Some created a central contract vehicle such as a physician hospital organization (PHO), which was owned or control-led by both the hospital and physicians seeking to contract with managed care plans on behalf of each of the hospital and physicians. Others created a management service organization (MSO), which would provide the services of the PHO and also other management services to the physician group and possibly the hospital.

Many moved to more fully integrated delivery systems wherein the physician and hospital component were part of one corporate entity or series of related corporate entities. The development of the IDS might be accomplished by a number of methods, including the creation of a nonprofit medical foundation, the purchase of physi-cian assets by the foundation or a hospital or its related organization, or through the employment of physicians. Individual physicians and physician groups consolidated, merged, and sought affiliations with other physicians and physician groups to expand, and develop a greater capacity and ability to participate in managed care contracting. Hospital systems also consolidated, merged, and sought affiliations with other hospitals to maximize their ability to participate in the managed care market and to network and affiliate with physician groups. Managed care organizations also began to consolidate, merge, and seek affiliations. Many sought to develop stronger relationships with physicians to the exclusion of hospitals. Others sought to become part of systems which included hospitals.

With the dynamic movement to managed care and the proliferation of integrated delivery systems to assist in the management of such care, the stage was set for one of the greatest revolutions in healthcare in the United States.

2

Types of Managed Care Organizations and Products

HEALTH MAINTENANCE ORGANIZATIONS (HMOs)

Health maintenance organizations (HMOs) are entities which receive premium payments from an employer group, other entity, or an individual with the understanding that the HMO will be financially responsible for all the healthcare required by an enrollee for a specified period of time provided through the HMO's provider networks. The HMO typically develops a provider network by contracting with physicians, hospitals, and other providers and suppliers to ensure adequate healthcare coverage for its enrollees. The HMO's enrollees are required to obtain their care through the provider network, except for certain out-of-area and emergency care. The HMO may employ certain providers and own certain provider entities. The HMO assumes the risk that the amount paid by the employer group or individuals will cover the cost of treatment by the providers and suppliers in the system. As a risk-bearing entity, it is generally licensed as an HMO either by a State Department of Insurance or Corporations. It may be licensed separately from an indemnity insurer, and it must meet numerous state requirements with respect to solvency, reserves, and provider networks. A patient usually chooses a primary care physician in the HMO as his or her physician. A patient who does not chose a physician may remain unassigned for a period of time or be assigned to a primary care physician. The physician typically acts as a gatekeeper, and the patient must first visit or contact the primary care physician to obtain a referral to visit another physician, such as a specialist. HMOs typically provide their physician services through an IPA, staff, group, or hybrid model.

IPA Model HMO

An independent practice association (IPA) consists of physicians who have not commingled their assets and liabilities into one entity and are not practicing in a truly integrated fashion, but maintain their separate practices and participate in the IPA as a means to contract with HMOs or other health plans. Where IPAs primarily contract with the HMO to provide services to the HMO's members, the HMO model typically is called an IPA model HMO.

Staff Model HMO

In a staff model HMO, the physicians are employees of the HMO or provide substantially all their physician services to HMO members pursuant to direct contracts with the HMO. This latter alternative generally is found in states where HMOs cannot employ physicians. The physicians in the staff model HMO typically do not render services to other HMOs or health plans.

Group Model HMO

A group model HMO has a contract with one or more medical groups to provide all the necessary services to the HMO's enrollees. The medical groups may be primary care, specialty based, and/or multi-specialty in nature. Such medical groups are typically integrated: the physicians have commingled all their assets, liabilities, and practices at one or more predominant sites and possibly at satellite locations. The medical groups generally are not exclusive to any one HMO, and thus they provide physician services for more than one HMO, for other health plans, and to self-pay patients.

Some medical groups may not have transferred all the assets and liabilities of the physicians to one entity, but only achieved partial integration of the practices. In addition, the physicians may transfer much of their assets and liabilities to the new entity, but continue to practice in a number of independent offices without one main site and satellite offices. This structure is often called a clinic without walls (CWW), or group practice without walls (GPWW), because the physicians are part of one organizational entity, but are practicing in separate locations. The HMO also could contract with such a group to provide services to the HMO's beneficiaries.

Hybrid Model HMOs

Hybrid models exist. For example, to obtain necessary physician coverage, an HMO might contract with both a number of IPAs and medical groups and may even employ physicians in some areas. What is most important to the HMO is that it develop a base of cost-effective providers who can manage care. As a result, the physician model for the HMO may differ in certain localities, although to the extent possible, an HMO might want to develop some consistency in its provider networks.

HMO Contracts with Hospitals

Unless the HMO owns hospitals, it must contract with a series of hospital providers to ensure hospital coverage for its enrollees. Typically, the HMO negotiates contract rates with hospitals which depend upon the nature of the market, the competition, and other facts and circumstances. The HMO will want to contract with hospitals which are cost-effective, to ensure that the HMO's costs are reasonable and its premiums competitive.

PREFERRED PROVIDER ORGANIZATIONS (PPOs)

A preferred provider organization (PPO) typically contracts on behalf of employer groups or other plans with hospital and physician providers at reduced rates. The hospitals and physicians who become part of the preferred provider network generally are either called preferred or participating providers. As discussed above, generally there is an incentive to the patient to utilize a preferred provider. Thus, a patient who visits a physician who is not a preferred provider likely will have to pay a higher copayment or deductible. Providers offer discounts to PPOs in anticipation of achieving additional patient volumes, or to minimize the chances that their patient volume will go to another provider.

PPOs do not assume financial risk in the same manner as HMOs. As a result, the licensing provisions applicable to HMOs typically do not apply to PPOs, although there can be state licensing laws or other regulatory provisions affecting PPOs.

Messenger PPOs

Many preferred provider organizations merely act as messengers. That is, the PPO acts on behalf of a payor, but the PPO does not intend to assume any obligations to pay the hospital or physician preferred providers. The providers should know on whose behalf the PPO is purporting to act, and ascertain sufficient background information concerning the payor, to enable it to determine whether the provider wants to enter into the arrangement with the PPO. The PPO may collect its fee as a percentage of the discount it has obtained for the payor.

In some messenger arrangements, a contract between the payor and the provider is executed, and in other instances, one is not. In the former situation, the PPO tenders the contractual arrangement between the payor and the provider to each entity, and both the payor and the provider execute it, or the PPO has been designated by the payors as their attorney-in-fact to execute such agreements on their behalf. In the latter instance, there is no privity of contract between the provider and the payor, and the provider remains at substantial financial risk. It must rely on the PPO's declaration that the payor *should* pay the provider, unless the payor will execute a document incorporating the terms and conditions of the PPO's contract with the provider, and either have the provider execute it or make it a third-party beneficiary of the agreement.

It is unclear why providers would enter into arrangements with PPOs where there is no direct agreement with the payor requiring that the payor pay the provider, or an attorney-in-fact arrangement. One can assume that competitive marketplace pressures or the clout of the PPO might be the reason.

Direct PPO Contracts

Sometimes PPOs operate on their own behalf and assume the payment obligation to the providers. At least in these latter instances, a provider should know with whom it is contracting and that there will be privity of contract. However, the provider should ascertain as much information as possible about the PPO, its financial conditions, and its operations to ensure that it is not contracting with a shell or thinly capitalized entity which might not be able to stand by its promise to pay the provider.

EXCLUSIVE PROVIDER ORGANIZATIONS

Exclusive provider organizations (EPOs), as noted above, are entities which create exclusive provider networks in which a beneficiary can access the system only through the providers who are part of that system. The lack of flexibility in many EPO systems has, in part, resulted in their limited popularity.

HEALTHCARE SERVICE PLANS

Healthcare service plans, typically operated by Blue Cross and Blue Shield Plans throughout the country, have provided healthcare coverage for many years. Although initially they acted like indemnity carriers, merely paying claims, many began to develop managed care products to compete with companies offering HMO, PPO, and EPO products, although not necessarily through the same corporate entities which operate the healthcare service plans.

THIRD-PARTY ADMINISTRATORS (TPAs) AND ADMINISTRATIVE SERVICES ORGANIZATIONS (ASOs)

Many self-insured groups, such as employers and union trusts, will use third-party administrators (TPAs) or administrative services organizations (ASOs) to manage and pay their claims. In lieu of paying premiums to health insurers who would charge group premiums to pay for the healthcare services rendered to the group's beneficiaries, these self-insured groups assume the risk of the provision of such services on their own, possibly with some stop loss insurance. The self-insured group may contract directly with providers, and it may use the services of a PPO. TPAs and ASOs are neither health plans nor insurers, but entities which provide claims-paying functions for the entities which they service. Although historically such entities merely paid claims, their functions have expanded. Many have some function in the management of care. In addition, many self-insured groups were pioneers in PPO development, and thus a TPA or ASO may be paying claims based on discounted rates negotiated by a PPO on behalf of a self-insured group.

Stop loss insurance is insurance which can be purchased to pay or assist in the payment of a healthcare claim if it exceeds a certain amount. With respect to a self-insured group, if the charges or payments associated with a particular patient exceed a certain amount, *e.g.*, $100,000 or $250,000, the stop loss insurance will pay the amount over the threshold amount, provided the group has purchased the appropriate stop loss policy.

SINGLE OR SPECIALTY SERVICE PLANS

There also are single or specialty service plans, such as health plans which provide services only in the mental health area, or vision and dental plans. Mental health plans developed as a recognition grew that a carve-out of mental health services might stem the rate of increases in costs for mental healthcare and facilitate the management of such care. Employer groups could contract with these specialty health plans for services which focus on mental health. Vision and dental plans have often been add-on or supplemental coverage to health plans. They vary greatly in the benefits and services that they offer, and represent another example of single or specialty service plans.

HMO-LIKE ORGANIZATIONS AND PRODUCTS
PPOs Using a Gatekeeper

The distinctions between many of the managed care organizations and products have become blurred. Many PPOs now employ the gatekeeper concept by ensuring that each enrollee chooses a primary care physician. PPOs determined that merely obtaining discounts from providers was insufficient to keep their costs of providing care from increasing at substantial rates. As a result, PPOs began to look at more ways to manage care; one way included the requirement that each PPO patient choose a primary care physician or that the PPO assign such a physician to the patient.

The primary care physician must authorize certain services, and make referrals to a specialist within the preferred provider network if the patient is to be subject to the lower copayment. There can be a significant difference between what a patient pays for a visit to a preferred provider, with the proper authorization or referral, and what the patient pays to visit a nonpreferred physician without an appropriate referral. As a result, for financial reasons, many patients are forced to use the preferred provider network, which is where the PPO can truly attempt to contain costs and manage care.

Point of Service Plans

HMOs have developed certain PPO options to enable their patients to visit other physicians. A point-of-service (POS) plan, for instance, allows a beneficiary to elect at the time of service whether to access the HMO benefits and thus visit an HMO provider, access the PPO benefits and thus visit a preferred provider, or go out of network and pay the higher deductible and copayment. Where there are three such options, the plan might be known as a triple option plan. Inasmuch as POS plans typically include an HMO option, the entity offering this option must be a licensed HMO or insurer or have an agreement whereby such services are offered through the HMO.

MEDICARE RISK PLANS

Medicare risk plans began to proliferate after the middle 1980s with a change in the federal requirements for HMOs which enroll Medicare patients. Such plans receive a portion of the money which the Medicare program would have spent on healthcare coverage for the Medicare beneficiaries and offer an HMO package of benefits to the Medicare beneficiaries at a reduced out-of-pocket cost to them. These products offered by health plans are often known as Seniors Plans. To participate in the Medicare Risk program, an entity has to be a federally qualified HMO or a Competitive Medical Plan approved as such by the Medicare program.

MEDICAID RISK PLANS

Many Medicaid plans have shifted to a form of managed care by employing a greater use of HMO or HMO-like products. Inasmuch as Medicaid programs typically have not covered much preventative care and their payments to physicians have been low, when a state develops a Medicaid managed care product, it often can provide care to Medicaid beneficiaries in a more cost-effective manner because the beneficiaries receive preventative care and visit a physician sooner. The Medicaid beneficiary is not relegated to accessing medical care through the emergency department of the hospital.

INDEMNITY PLANS

Although many indemnity plans continue to exist, they generally are not viewed as managed care organizations. They indemnify the patient or subscriber for the healthcare services which the patient has obtained. Usually, the indemnity carrier will pay the provider directly where the patient has assigned his or her benefits to the indemnity carrier. Many of the indemnity carriers which remain often have attempted to include PPO-like characteristics to reduce their costs.

CONCLUSION

There are myriad managed care organizations and products. Their distinctions are increasingly becoming blurred as managed care organizations seek to differentiate their products in the marketplace and offer employer groups and consumers products which they desire.

3

Forms of
Provider Payment

HOSPITAL PAYMENTS

Hospitals are reimbursed by health plans in a variety of ways. As discussed above, with the development of HMOs, many hospital providers initially were paid their billed charges for services rendered to HMO patients, and the HMOs sought to manage the utilization of hospital services. As PPOs began to proliferate, discounting became more common.

Percentage Discounts from Charges

When HMOs first sought discounts from hospital charges, many hospitals offered them, typically in the form of percentage discounts. Such discounts had the advantage of being easy to calculate, but they did not result in much cost containment because a hospital might merely increase its charges. Occasionally, health plans sought to limit a hospital's increase in its charges to preclude a hospital from increasing the charges to make up for any discount. Many health plans, *e.g.*, Blue Cross and Blue Shield plans, had other mechanisms for paying providers, such as a cost- or fee-schedule basis. Inasmuch as the payments to hospitals on such a basis might be settled yearly through some reporting mechanism, the hospitals might be paid a

Periodic Interim Payment (PIP), almost as a form of interim or current financing to ensure that the hospitals received some form of payment prior to settlement.

Per Diem Payments

In the early 1980s, per diem payments to hospitals—a fixed amount per day per patient—became a popular means by which health plans would compensate hospitals for inpatient hospital care. With a per diem payment, all the costs associated with a patient's stay in the hospital, including the use of the emergency department prior to admission, supplies, equipment, hospital room, and hospital costs associated with surgical procedures would be included in the per diem payment. Often, the costs associated with certain hospital-based physicians, such as emergency department physicians and pathologists, also were included in the per diem rate. The health plan, of course, would still seek to reduce the number of days for which a patient stayed in the hospital with the result that the health plan achieved savings from both paying on a per diem basis and the reduced number of days. How many per diem payments would be due to the hospital generally depended upon the number of days the patient was in the hospital at the census hour, the time at which the patient population was determined (generally at 12 midnight).

Stratified Per Diem Payments

Many per diem payment mechanisms were stratified; that is, the hospital might be paid one rate for a medical surgical day (a day when a patient was on the medical/surgical service), another rate for a critical care unit day (a day when a patient was in the critical care unit), a separate rate for an obstetrical day (a day when a patient was in the obstetrical unit), and any other iterations which made sense for the hospital, and to which the health plan agreed.

For example, a hospital would be paid three critical care unit per diems and two medical/surgical per diems for a patient who spent three days in the critical care unit and two days in the medical/surgical unit. Often, health plans sought to pay only one per diem for obstetrical patients who had delivered babies when those babies were in the nursery. However, health plans might pay an additional per diem rate if the newborn was in the neonatal intensive care unit (NICU) when the mother was in the hospital, or the newborn remained in the hospital after the mother was discharged. Such latter patients are typically called boarder babies. A plan may pay a separate NICU rate or a boarder baby rate if such separate rates were negotiated.

Extraordinary Payments outside the Per Diem

Hospitals also sought to negotiate extraordinary payment for certain types of services, supplies, or drugs when the hospital was being paid a per diem rate. For example, hospitals might receive separate, additional payments for certain orthotic supplies whose cost exceeded a certain amount or for very expensive drugs. The payment mechanism to the hospital for such supplies or drugs might be a percentage discount from charges, or more likely cost plus a small percentage markup. The cost of certain orthotics or drugs might exceed thousands of dollars, and for a short patient stay, the per diem payments would in no way cover these costs.

Case Rate or DRG Payments

Some hospitals began to negotiate case rates on the inpatient side. These case rates might be the same amount for any case, differing amounts for differing cases, or DRG payments. The payment would cover the entire course of treatment in the hospital.

Global or Package Pricing

Hospitals even began to offer global or package pricing, which included a price for a basket of services, *e.g.*, a course of rehabilitation treatment or cardiovascular surgery. These payments rates might even include all or part of the physician's component of providing the care during the hospital inpatient stay.

Outpatient Discounts from Charges

When many hospitals first negotiated per diem arrangements with health plans on the inpatient side, the outpatient services were paid at a discount from charges. Occasionally, the discounted charge for an outpatient procedure might exceed the per diem rate which would be payable to the hospital if the patient was an inpatient, particularly if the patient received an ambulatory surgical procedure. Hospitals sought to be paid at the discounted rate for such ambulatory procedures, and health plans occasionally tried to limit the payment to a per diem amount.

Outpatient Fee Schedules

It generally was thought that the inpatient component of hospital services was so great that it was the main area of focus. However, as more and more procedures continually shifted to the outpatient area, health plans sought outpatient fee schedules for services rendered by hospitals, particularly for ambulatory surgical center services. Freestanding ambulatory surgery centers provided much competition to hospitals in this area, and because of their lower cost structure, both in cost of facilities and personnel, were generally able to provide ambulatory surgical services at a much lower cost than hospital facilities. Such freestanding centers accepted payment rates based on fee schedules, exerting pressure on hospitals to accept fee schedule payments for ambulatory surgical services which could be provided in the freestanding setting.

Stop Loss Payments

As part of many of these discounted arrangements, hospitals sought to negotiate stop loss (or reinsurance) coverage, which would provide a hospital additional payments for services rendered to a patient, where the costs or charges associated with treating a patient exceeded a certain amount. For example, if the hospital's charges associated with treating a particular patient exceed $50,000, a hospital might be paid based on a percentage discount from its charges for the amount over $50,000 or for the entire amount, depending on the nature of the agreement it reached for stop loss coverage.

Capitation Payments

Hospitals also negotiated capitated payment arrangements with health plans. In such payment systems, a hospital would be paid a fixed amount per member per month for all hospital services which might be needed by an HMO's enrollees. The capitation payment might be age/sex adjusted for the patient population for which the hospital would be responsible. There might be stop loss payments available to the hospital if it "purchased" stop loss insurance from the HMO, and the capitated payment might not cover out-of-area emergency care. The risk relationships established through capitation could be on a shared, partial, or full risk basis.

Shared Risk

In a typical shared risk situation, the hospital might be paid currently on a per diem or other basis, but the amount of money it is ultimately paid would be based on a capitated amount which was put in a risk pool. If hospital utilization was low and there were monies left in the risk pool, the hospital might share the monies remaining in the risk pool with the health plan and/or physicians. Monies might be left in the risk pool after paying the hospital and any other providers or suppliers the hospital was obligated to pay. The contractors to the hospital incur charges or costs for the provision of services or supplies to beneficiaries, for which the hospital is financially responsible. Before these charges or costs are reported by the provider or supplier to the hospital, they are called "incurred but not reported" amounts (IBNRs).

In a shared risk arrangement, the hospital might only share in the upside risk. That is, the hospital could receive additional monies from the risk pool because of low utilization, but it would not be sharing in the downside risk. Thus, if utilization was high, the hospital would not have to pay money back to the health plan. Although, as utilization increased, there might be a mechanism in the agreement with the hospital to withhold more of its payments until utilization decreased.

Partial Risk

In a partial risk relationship, the hospital typically shares in both the upside and downside risk, but it is not required to pay any amounts beyond what is provided for in the risk pools, as would be the case in the full risk situation. It is particularly important for hospitals which assume partial or full risk need to have mechanisms in place which permit them to manage care efficiently and economically.

Full Risk

In a full risk capitation situation, the hospital would be at full risk for rendering all the services to which it had contractually committed. It might participate in some form of a risk pool to facilitate the alignment of incentives, but the hospital would be at full risk, and if money was not available in any risk pool to pay for the other services, the hospital would have to pay it out of its operating funds or reserves.

Percentage of Health Plan Premiums

As discussed above, certain hospitals also sought to obtain a percentage of health plan premiums. Often health plans are reluctant to pay hospitals on such a basis because it may affect their ability to provide the administrative services which they believe are necessary to control costs and manage a system, and it leads to questions as to the true role of the health plans. However, larger provider systems often are interested in assuming some of the functions of the health plans.

Ambulatory Payment Groups (APGs)

An emerging payment alternative is payment based on ambulatory payment groups. In such a payment system, a patient is described by APGs that correspond to each service which has been provided to the patient. Multiple APGs may be assigned to each patient. APGs take into account the diversity of sites in which services can be rendered. There are standard payment rates associated with each APG. Payment for services to a patient is determined by summing the payment rates across all APGs which have been assigned to the patient. However, to encourage efficiencies, certain procedures are consolidated, ancillaries are packaged, and the payment is discounted for multiple significant procedures and ancillaries. The Medicare program is considering implementing APGs for the outpatient technical component in the near future.

PHYSICIAN PAYMENTS

Physician payment by health plans on a capitated basis, and the health plans' movement to capitation payments for physicians, has been much more dramatic than that of hospitals. In the 1970s and early 1980s, when HMOs often were paying hospitals their billed charges for hospital services, physicians typically were not being paid their billed charges by health plans, unless there were no other physicians in the area providing that type of service with a discount.

Discount from Charges and Fee Schedule Payments

Physicians typically agreed to discounts from their charges for health plans either through percentage discounts from charges or the acceptance of certain fee schedule payments by health plans which have resulted in payment of less than the physicians' charge schedules. In fact, the Medicare program now pays physicians according to a Resource Based Relative Value Scale (RBRVS) payment schedule.

Case Rates and Global or Package Pricing Arrangements

In addition, physicians also have negotiated case rates and global or package pricing arrangements. Case rates compensate physicians one amount for a course of treatment or procedure. Health plans might negotiate a case rate with physicians for a rehabilitation treatment plan for a patient or for a surgical procedure. Global or package pricing arrangements have become more common for cardiovascular surgery and certain other procedures which can easily be packaged by physicians into one price for a bundle of services. With respect to cardiovascular surgery, a health plan might make one payment to the heart surgery team for the physician component of heart surgery, and that payment would have to cover all the physician services associated with the heart surgery. A further packaged price might be developed for the physician and the hospital components of cardiac surgery.

Many health plans are particularly interested in reducing their costs for high priced specialty surgical procedures. Patients generally are willing to travel further to obtain those procedures, and thus a health plan may have more negotiating ability with the providers offering such services. As a result, the health plan can achieve lower prices, thus reducing its costs.

Capitation Payments

Physicians have accepted and managed capitation on a shared risk, partial risk, and full risk basis much more than hospital providers. They have been particularly interested in obtaining age/sex adjusted capitation rates for the patient populations for which they are responsible. Such adjustment mechanisms are particularly important for a primary care pediatrician who might have a disproportionate number of patients who are under two years of age. These younger patients utilize a significant amount of healthcare resources and receive numerous vaccinations and well-baby care.

It was generally thought easier to manage the physician services within a budget than managing the hospital's costs. The reason for this assumption may be that physicians have more experience in managing care and capitation than hospitals. Typically, however, the cost of a hospital stay would far exceed the professional fee to be paid to the physicians rendering services at the hospital. When many physician providers began to move toward capitation in the early 1980s, many hospitals were paid on a per diem basis by health plans. By keeping utilization of hospital services down, the physicians often shared the upside potential in a risk pool with the health plan. Increasingly, both physicians and hospitals are seeking to incur greater risk under capitation contracts and to manage the care on their own, in an attempt to gain control over their destinies and manage more of the healthcare dollars in the system.

Percentage of Premiums

Physicians also are seeking percentage of premium payments. As with hospitals, managed care plans are often reluctant to provide physicians with a percentage of the health plan premium, thus decreasing the need for the health plan services and their usefulness in the healthcare system.

Ambulatory Payment Groups

APGs might be implemented for physician services on the commercial side as an alternative to capitation.

ANCILLARY PROVIDER PAYMENTS
Modified Fee-for-Service or Fee Schedule Payments

Although hospital and physician payments represent the largest amount of payments by health plans for healthcare services rendered to enrollees, payments also are made to ancillary providers such as laboratories, pharmacies, home health agencies, and allied health practitioners. The form of compensation to these ancillary providers can vary substantially. If the health plan is paying the ancillary providers directly, often the payments are made on a modified fee-for-service or fee schedule basis.

Capitated Payments

Capitated payments are sometimes made to ancillary service providers. Such capitated payments may be made by the health plan or another provider. Often, the health plan will pay two capitated rates —one to the hospital and one to the physicians—and either group might be capitated for the services of the ancillary providers. That group will then seek to enter into contracts with the ancillary service providers. If there is a sufficient number of lives to reduce the risk to an ancillary service provider of agreeing to a capitation payment, the hospital or physician group might subcapitate the ancillary service providers. If there is not a sufficient number of lives, the hospital or physician group likely will have to pay the ancillary service provider on a modified fee-for-service basis.

Ancillary service providers which contract with health plans, medical groups, or hospitals on a capitated basis must be careful to ensure that the delivery system affords them appropriate utilization controls. An ancillary service provider such as a laboratory or pharmacy will not want to be put at risk for providing all tests or drugs which might be ordered by physicians unless it has some assurance that the physician will order only appropriate tests and pharmaceuticals in a cost-effective manner.

Hospital's Desire to Provide Ancillary Services on Behalf of Physicians

Obviously, if the physicians are capitated for ancillary services such as outpatient radiology, laboratory, and certain ambulatory surgery center services, they will seek to purchase these services at the lowest possible rate. Often the hospital at which the physicians practice will want to make the services available for the physicians on a subcontract basis. The physicians' willingness to contract with a hospital in such instances will depend upon a hospital's ability to competitively price its services. However, a hospital may face myriad legal issues in such discount paying arrangements.

For example, the amount of the discount offered to the physicians by the hospital might be viewed by the Office of the Inspector General of the Department of Health and Human Services as a disguised payment for the referral of Medicare and Medicaid patients by the physicians, and thus in contravention of the Medicare and Medicaid antikickback laws. If the payment rates offered by the hospital are lower than those offered to the Medicare or Medicaid programs, the hospital might be seen as reducing its charges for such services; and those programs may argue that the reduced charges should be passed on to the Medicare and Medicaid programs, and the failure to do so is in violation of the Medicare and Medicaid false claims laws. If the hospital is tax-exempt and the rate at which it offers the services to the physicians is below fair market value or what is commercially reasonable, there might be allegations that the hospital is violating the prohibition against inurement of benefit, and its tax-exempt status could be adversely affected.

An additional consideration for the physicians and the hospital has to be the rate at which another provider or supplier might provide the service. It may be that the cost structure of such other providers or suppliers is so much lower than the hospital that the hospital cannot effectively compete. In addition, the hospital may find itself in a quandary with respect to the provision of such services to the physicians. It may be required to provide the services at a very low price to be competitive with the other ancillary providers and suppliers, but doing so may subject the hospital to some of the legal risks mentioned above because the price offered to the physicians might be seen as too low by the government regulators.

Although at first glance the hospital might be able to minimize these allegations if it offers such services on a capitated basis, it is possible that such an offer also may be scrutinized on the above lines, and it may also be questionable in some states as to whether a hospital, on behalf of the physicians, could assume such financial risk for doing so.

An often overlooked consideration of a hospital providing such discounted ancillary services is the possibility that the physicians might share these rates with the health plans with which the hospital contracts. Their motivation for doing so might be financially based where the hospital is paid on a modified fee-for-service basis by the health plan for such ancillaries, but the use of ancillaries is subject to a risk pool which the physicians share in if the use and cost of those ancillaries is low. Of course, a hospital will want to ensure that any arrangements for ancillary services which it might have with its physicians are kept confidential.

PROPERLY ACCOUNTING FOR PAYMENTS

As noted above, there are myriad payment relationships providers can enter into with health plans. To the extent that those payment relationships deviate from the standard payment mechanisms which the plans have with other providers, the provider with the differing payment arrangement must pay particular attention to whether it is actually being paid in accordance with the agreement. Thus, the provider should have a monitoring system in place to determine whether it is being paid consistent with the terms of the agreement.

Similarly, a health plan should not agree to a payment mechanism unless it can actually pay the provider in accordance with such mechanism. Occasionally, in both parties' zeal to agree on a mutually acceptable payment mechanism, they will agree to a payment system which the health plan's information system cannot account for absent some manual adjustment, and the provider has no system in place to determine whether it is being paid consistent with the agreed upon manner.

For example, the parties may agree that the health plan will pay the provider's cost of administering the drug AZT plus a markup of 5%. Unless the provider indicates in some manner its cost of AZT, not its charges, and the 5% markup, the health plan would not know what to pay. Even if the provider did properly indicate its costs on its bill to the health plan for the AZT, the health plan's information system might not understand the provider's bill and/or pay in accordance with the bill. Finally, once the provider has been paid, it will have to be able to properly monitor the health plan's payment of its bill.

CONCLUSION

There are many forms of provider payment, from percentage discounts from charges and fee schedules to per diem payments, case rates or DRG payments, and global or package pricing. Capitation payments, however, are becoming increasingly accepted and desired, and many providers seek to be paid on a percentage of premium basis.

4

Capitation as a Preferred Payment Mechanism

NEED TO ALIGN INCENTIVES

Any payment system which does not align the incentives of the providers in that system will not be successful in maintaining costs to the lowest extent possible. If a hospital is being paid a fixed amount per day for each day a patient is in the hospital and the physician attending the patient is being paid a fixed amount per month for treating the patient, the incentives in the system are not aligned. The hospital wants the patient to stay longer; the physician wants the patient to be discharged earlier.

Conversion of the hospital to a DRG system, where the hospital is paid a flat rate per admission, does not solve the problem because although the hospital is incentivized to discharge the patient sooner, it still has the incentive to have the patient admitted to the hospital and the physician has the incentive not to admit the patient.

Of course, one can suggest that health plan preauthorization, continued stay, and retrospective reviews could ensure that the system will work, but health plan authorization and reviews do not align incentives and they involve significant administrative time and expense. It appears that incentives are best aligned in a manner which is consistent with cost containment when both parties, the hospital and the physicians, are working toward the same goal, wellness of the patient, and they are both subject to a system which pays a fixed amount per member per month. This is not to suggest, however, that physicians in the medical group, the physician practice division, or physician employees have to be paid in a capitated manner on an individual basis, or that all physicians should be capitated. However, in the aggregate, they should be paid on a capitated basis.

MINIMUM NUMBER OF CAPITATED LIVES

For capitation to have a chance at being successful, a system must have some minimum number of capitated lives over which to spread the risk. The number of lives for which a primary care physician should be responsible is substantially less than the number of lives for which a gastroenterologist or an orthopedic surgeon should be responsible. And the number of lives for which the gastroenterologist or orthopedic surgeon should be responsible should be substantially less than the number of lives for which a cardiovascular surgeon or neurosurgeon should be responsible. The reason, of course, is that the incidence of an individual visiting a gastroenterologist or orthopedic surgeon is substantially less than the incidence of someone visiting a primary care physician, and likewise with respect to cardiovascular surgeons or neurosurgeons in comparison to gastroenterologists or orthopedic surgeons.

PRIMARY CARE PHYSICIANS
(PCPs) AS GATEKEEPERS

Primary care physicians (PCPs) are at the focal point of any capitated system. They are the gatekeepers. An enrollee chooses a primary care physician from a list of the PCPs who have contracted with the health plan. Generally, the PCP is part of a larger medical group or integrated delivery system (see Chapters 7 and 8). A PCP will want to have enough lives under capitation and at high enough rates that he or she can make a comfortable living without substantial risk.

As a general rule, the more lives the PCP has under capitation, the less chance that the PCP will experience a disproportionate number of sick enrollees. An individual PCP who is not part of a medical group which has many PCPs with enrollees under capitation can be at greater risk because he or she faces a greater prospect of having to be responsible for a disproportionate amount of very ill enrollees. As the number of capitated lives and PCPs in the group increases, the risk is diminished because of the numbers. That is, with more enrollees, the incidence of disease and illness is more predictable and can be accounted for with greater certainty.

Physicians, of course, can buy stop loss insurance which might insure them against the charges for a specific enrollee exceeding a certain amount in a particular year, *e.g.*, $25,000, $50,000, or $100,000. Stop loss insurance, however, is not inexpensive. As a result, the more lives a group has under capitation, the higher is the threshold for which it might purchase stop loss insurance and the lower its costs might be for stop loss insurance.

Often the health plan retains part of the capitation payment to the PCP or pays a lesser capitated amount to account for the payments to providers who are out of the service area and/or for emergencies. Obviously, a provider would not be able to anticipate all the out-of-area providers its enrollees may have to visit or the emergency situations which might arise, but actuarial calculations are made to estimate these costs.

SUBCAPITATION OF SPECIALISTS VS. MODIFIED FEE-FOR-SERVICE PAYMENTS

Initially, many people thought that merely capitating the PCPs would contain the costs in the system and lead to the necessary alignment of incentives. They believed that the specialists should continue to be paid on a fee-for-service basis. Such a notion, however, is no longer as well accepted; many believe, in fact, it is incorrect. If the PCPs receive the original source capitation payment—that is, a capitation payment directly from the health plan—and they are responsible for paying for all other physician services and certain ancillary services, the real financial risk to the PCP is in these payments which the PCPs might have to make to the specialists, subspecialists, and the ancillary providers.

A PCP capitated by a health plan for primary care only, might have to work harder by having more patient encounters and ordering a few more laboratory tests. A PCP capitated for all physician services and certain ancillaries assumes the risk of overutilization by specialists, subspecialists, and ancillary providers unless they also receive capitation payments or are subject to some overall aggregate payment limitation. If the PCPs are at risk for overutilization by the specialists, subspecialists, and ancillary providers, the risk may be significant.

The specialists and the subspecialists order the expensive tests and perform the costly procedures. They generally seem to prefer to be paid on a modified fee-for-service basis. Many view their participation in managed care on a fee-for-service basis as retaining some semblance of their former practices. Absent any withholds which would put some of the specialists' or subspecialists' compensation at risk, a PCP paying a specialist or a subspecialist on a modified fee-for-service basis has little control over utilization once he or she makes the referral.

The parties often seek to reduce the modified fee-for-service payment of the specialists or subspecialists at the outset by placing a portion of it in a risk pool. If the utilization does not exceed a certain amount, all or part of the monies in the risk pool may be returned to the specialists.

To fully align the incentives of the system, however, and to reduce the risk to the PCPs, it may be preferable to capitate the specialists and the subspecialists in the system. Such capitation might be accomplished by the health plan paying the specialists and subspecialists on a capitated basis, or more appropriately, the PCPs paying the specialists and the subspecialists a subcapitated rate. Of course, the parties will want to ensure that the system employs

certain utilization controls to preclude the PCPs from merely referring all cases to specialists.

OBSTACLES TO IMPLEMENTING
SPECIALTY CAPITATION

Specialty capitation is much more difficult to institute successfully
than PCP capitation. There are two principal reasons: (1) the number
of lives which must be assigned to make it advantageous for a
specialist to contract on a capitated basis is much greater than the
number of lives required by the PCP; and (2) the incidence of a
disproportionately ill patient population can be much more trouble-
some to a specialist, who might have to perform costly procedures
and order expensive tests than to a primary care physician who might
only need to have a few additional office visits with the patient.

It is important to note, however, that if PCPs are responsible for
specialty care because they are paying specialists on a modified
fee-for-service basis, the PCPs assume the risks for services they
cannot control and cannot even provide. As a result, it is important
in the success of any system to align incentives by making the
specialists and subspecialists responsible for the medical care which
is within their control.

Specialty physicians are often less willing than PCPs to accept
capitation because it is often difficult to ensure that there will be
enough lives assigned to specialists to make it worth their while in
assuming the risk of providing the specialty care. For example, if an
eye physician is capitated at $0.60 per member per month, it would
take 10,000 lives assigned to that eye physician for the physician to
be paid only $6,000 per month. If a few of these lives required major
surgery in a month, the eye physician could be at a loss for the
month.

One factor in favor of the PCPs in trying to enlist the services of
specialists on a capitated basis is the excess of specialists in the United
States and in most major market areas. As a result, where there is an
excess of specialists, it is much easier for PCPs to convince the

specialists to accept capitation because they fear that their physician competitors may do so to their exclusion. It also is possible for specialists to contract with a number of PCP groups and/or systems to ensure that they have sufficient lives under capitation to reduce the risk.

Although specialty and subspecialty capitation is probably the best way to ensure the alignment of incentives among the physicians, the hospital, and the system, a system must have a substantial number of lives (*e.g.*, over a couple hundred thousand and in some cases 500,000 to 1,000,000) in order to capitate all specialists and subspecialists. The incidence of the need for bone marrow transplant physicians, pediatric neurosurgeons, and other superspecialty physicians providing quaternary care is so small that the number of lives necessary under capitation to ensure that such a specialist would provide services on a capitated basis is too great for most systems. As a result, many specialty physicians will have to remain on a modified fee-for-service basis. However, there should be strict utilization controls in the areas in which they practice.

FOCUS ON MAJOR SPECIALTY SERVICES

It is most important to capitate specialists and subspecialists for those services which are most often needed by the patient population. If the major services costing the bulk of the money are capitated, the risk can be reduced substantially, costs contained, and incentives aligned as best as possible. It also is important to note that before visiting one of these superspecialty physicians, who might be paid on a modified fee-for-service basis, the enrollee has most probably seen at least one other specialist in addition to the primary care physician. It also can be helpful to arrange a payment agreement with the superspecialist which might be in the form of some kind of package pricing, *e.g.*, a set amount per bone marrow transplant or payment by APGs. Further, there is probably less risk of unnecessary pediatric neurosurgical procedures than radiology procedures. In addition, it may be financially beneficial to purchase stop loss insurance at some threshold amount which might often be triggered by the high cost of some of the procedures performed by the superspecialists performing services on a modified fee-for-service basis.

ADVERSE SELECTION

There is at least one important caveat to capitating PCPs. If a PCP has a particular degree of expertise in treating a certain type of patient, such as patients who are HIV positive, and the PCP is located in an area where there are many HIV positive individuals, that PCP will most likely experience adverse selection. That is, many patients who have the propensity to be sicker than the average patient will choose such a physician as their PCP. A health plan or payment system needs to have a mechanism to adequately compensate such a physician or group for participation in the system beyond a standard capitation payment to ensure that such a physician will contract with the health plan and the services of that physician will be available to the health plan's enrollees. Often, physicians with such expertise can decrease the overall costs of treating such patients because of their special expertise.

SUBCAPITATION OF ANCILLARY SERVICES

As noted above, PCPs often are responsible for certain ancillary services. These services might include laboratory, pharmacy, home health, hospice, and/or ambulatory surgery center services. Of course, to the extent that the PCP can enter into capitated arrangements for such services, he or she can reduce his or her risks. However, strict utilization controls must be employed because a contracting laboratory or pharmacy which agrees to provide laboratory services or pharmaceuticals to a system on a capitated basis will want to ensure that the physician will not merely order more tests and drugs because they have subcapitated these ancillary services.

Home health and hospice services also can be capitated with the proper utilization controls. Ambulatory surgery center services also might be capitated. There is generally less concern with overutilization of ambulatory surgery center services than laboratory tests and pharmaceuticals because it is generally thought that the incidence of unnecessary surgeries is less than that of the incidence of ordering of unnecessary laboratory tests or pharmaceuticals.

THE TRANSITIONAL PERIOD TO CAPITATION

It is important to note that very few systems are 100% capitated. As a result, as systems move toward capitation, there remains a significant transitional period. For this transitional period, there often are not enough capitated lives to capitate most specialists, and there may not even be enough lives to capitate any of the specialists. As a result, payment mechanisms for this transitional phase must be employed. The best payment mechanisms are those which seek to align incentives as best as possible.

Some states may allow a risk pool where, although physicians are paid on modified fee-for-service basis, a portion of their payment is withheld and, if utilization is down, all or part of it is returned to them. Global or package pricing also might be employed. For example, for cardiovascular surgery, the chief surgeon may be paid a package price or global rate from which all other physicians on the surgical team must also be paid. Such pricing provides more certainty and makes possible greater cost containment. Another payment mechanism which might be useful in the transitional period and also aligns incentives is payment under AGPs. The PCP need not be as concerned when the patient is referred to the specialists if the specialist is being paid on an APG basis, and not a modified fee-for-service basis.

Finally, the hospital should be capitated for its services to ensure that the incentives of the parties are aligned. Unfortunately, hospitals have been late in coming to capitation. Many which participated in capitation contracts in the mid-1980s and earlier did not have the necessary safety mechanisms in place to monitor utilization and the necessary contractual arrangements to minimize the cost of the services for which they were financially responsible. Now, many health plans and physicians have recognized that much of the money in the system is contained in the hospital payment component, and if the hospital continues to be paid on a modified fee-for-service basis, the health plan and the physicians can realize greater revenues and profits by keeping hospital utilization down and not sharing the savings with the hospital.

Although this observation may be correct, it is important to realize that such a system makes it much more difficult to align the incentives of the hospital and the physicians. Of course, a risk pool arrangement might be employed, but the hospital must not only seek to get back its portion of the risk pool, but also contain costs to maximize its available capitated revenues. It is important to properly align the incentives of all the parties to contain costs and maintain quality care.

CAPITATION OF HOSPITALS AND SUBCONTRACTS

A better solution than refusing to capitate hospitals might be reducing somewhat the capitation payment to the hospital and sharing this difference with the health plans and the physicians up front. In fact some hospitals, in their zeal to become capitated providers, have done exactly that. Their reasoning is that they must learn how to manage care to a certain cost per member per month (pmpm); they do not want to have disincentives in their system to do so; and they want to capitalize on part of the revenues available through superior cost management rather than leaving all such monies for the health plans and the physicians.

As noted above, it is important for the PCPs who have contracted with health plans on a capitated basis to ensure that the medical and ancillary services which they cannot provide are provided in a cost-effective manner and at as little financial risk as possible to the PCP. This same analysis holds true for a hospital which is capitated. Unless a hospital can provide all the hospital services required by enrollees, it must have arrangements with other hospitals and possibly ancillary providers in the geographic areas where enrollees need any other services for which the hospital is capitated. These arrangements will most likely be on a modified fee-for-service basis where the hospital employs strict utilization controls.

Hospitals will want to assure that they obtain the best possible prices from other hospitals and ancillary providers. While it would likely be difficult for one hospital to subcapitate another in its service area because the originally capitated hospital will likely want to render any services on its premises, out-of-area hospitals might be subcapitated by the hospital or receive original source capitation payments directly from the health plan.

The nature of the hospital capitated will determine the nature of the relationship it has with other hospitals. If the hospital receiving the original source capitation payments from the health plan is a community hospital, it will likely have to contract with tertiary or quaternary facilities to provide that care for its enrollees. The tertiary facility with which the community hospital contracts might provide cardiovascular services, the quaternary facility might provide bone marrow transplantation services and gene therapy. The community hospital might also need to contract with other community hospitals if it is to provide services in a wide enough geographic area. If the community hospital is part of a hospital system with well placed hospitals, the hospital system might contract on behalf of the community hospital and other hospitals in the system.

If a tertiary or quaternary hospital holds the original source contract with the health plan, it might be able to provide all the services necessary for its enrollees, but it may not have the geographic coverage, and thus it might need to contract with other hospitals to ensure such geographic coverage. The tertiary facility may find it necessary to subcontract for superspecialty services with a quaternary or academic facility which can provide those services.

CONCLUSION

The alignment of incentives among the hospital and physician providers is not often easily accomplished. The labyrinth of relationships among the providers and the attendant compensation issues are significant. However, it is an important goal. Having the main components of the system—the physicians and the hospital—being paid on a capitated basis promotes such alignment because the parties are incentivized to keep the patient populations for which they are responsible well. They also are incentivized to manage and practice in a manner which minimizes costs pmpm and allocates resources in the best possible way. This drive toward capitation is leading to integrated delivery systems which assist the parties in taking and administering capitation (see Chapters 7 and 8).

It should be noted, however, that capitation to a PCP group may be very different from the compensation arrangement within such a group or within an integrated delivery system. That is, all the PCPs in a group or integrated delivery system may be capitated in the aggregate because the health plan pays a fixed amount pmpm multiplied by the number of members for which the PCPs are responsible. As a result, there is a fixed amount of money from which the PCPs can be paid. However, the PCPs or the integrated delivery system can arrange to compensate the individual PCPs within the system in whatever manner is deemed best.

Increasingly, although total compensation to the PCPs is limited by these total capitation payments, many PCPs are being paid for their patient encounters on a modified fee-for-service basis within their systems. Inasmuch as the PCPs do not order the most costly tests or perform the costly procedures, a PCP who has too many patient encounters merely works harder and sees more patients; he or she does not utilize many more resources. Thus, successful systems will likely be fully capitated, but the PCPs may be paid internally on a modified fee-for-service basis, the bulk of the specialists may be capitated, and the quaternary physicians paid on a global, package price basis or according to APGs. The total amount of money available to pay for physician services within the system, however, has been capitated by the health plan. In addition, the hospital is capitated with aligned incentives.

5

Managed Care Contracts and Terms

A managed care contract sets forth the nature and terms of the contractual relationship between the health plan and the provider. It is the document in which the parties evidence their agreement.

PARTIES TO THE CONTRACT

The managed care contract should set forth the parties to the contract. A provider contracting with the health plan should ask several questions. Who is the party with whom I am contracting? Is it a well-known insurance company or HMO, a thinly capitalized subsidiary, or a corporation merely related to another company which is known and respected? Is the health plan financially viable? What is its track record? If a vice-president for a major insurance company convinces a provider to sign a contract with a corporation merely related to the insurance company, absent some form of assumption of obligations or guarantee by the known insurance company, the provider merely has a contract with an unknown or little known entity.

The health plan also should ask some initial questions: Is this a new provider? Is it an IPA or a fully integrated medical group? How long has the provider been in existence? What is the provider's track record? Can the physicians comprising the provider or the hospital manage care? Will the physicians provide quality care? Is the provider appropriately licensed and certified?

DEFINITIONAL SECTION

There should be a definitional section in the contract which sets forth definitions for the most often used terms in the contract. Set forth below are four of the key definitions in a managed care contract, but all the definitions in that section should be read and understood by the provider.

Covered Services

This section might include a definition of covered services, *e.g.*, what services are covered by the health plan. This definition often includes a reference to those services which are set forth in individual benefit plans or those services which the health plan has agreed to make available for its beneficiaries. The provider should have access to a copy of each of the benefit plans which are within the scope of the contract, and possibly incorporate the benefit plans by reference into the contract. These plans are often updated, however, and the provider needs to ensure that it will be advised of such updates. This section is particularly important in a capitated contract where the provider has the obligation to provide such services for a fixed price. It is also important to determine whether an experimental or new service is included.

Medical Necessity

Contracts often define medical necessity, or such definitions are included in the benefit plans. A typical definition of medical necessity is:

> Services or supplies provided by a hospital, physician, or other provider that are required to identify or to treat an illness or injury and that are determined by the Plan to meet the following requirements:

1. Consistent with the symptoms or diagnosis and treatment of the condition, disease, ailment, or injury.

2. Appropriate with regard to standards of good medical practice.

3. Not solely for the convenience of the member, the physician, or other provider.

4. The most appropriate supply or level of service which can be safely provided to the member.

5. When applied to an inpatient, "medically necessary" means that the patient's symptoms or condition require services or supplies that cannot be safely provided to the patient as an outpatient.[1]

To the extent possible, a provider will want any definition of medical necessity to take into account the patient's condition at the time of rendering a service rather than a retrospective review. That is, although a health plan may retrospectively review whether the services rendered to a patient were medically necessary, they should be reviewed in the context of the patient's condition at the time he or she sought services.

Medical Emergency

Contracts will often define medical emergency. An emergency may be defined as follows: "A life-endangering illness which occurs suddenly and is severe enough to require immediate attention, and failure to provide such treatment could result in serious deterioration of the patient's condition or place the patient's life in jeopardy."[2] Providers should be careful to review any definition of emergency because health plans often seek to limit these definitions as much as possible, as services rendered in the event of emergency generally do not require preauthorization. Health plans do not want to pay for services as emergency services if they are not truly emergencies.

Eligibility

It also is important to define eligibility and how eligibility is determined. Providers want to be able to contact a health plan seven days a week, 24 hours a day to obtain current eligibility information, or even to be on line with respect to such information. Providers want to be able to conclusively rely on the eligibility information provided to them by a health plan, to ensure that if they provide services the health plan will not later refuse to pay based on the fact that the patient was ineligible to receive such services. Eligibility issues may arise for a number of reasons: for instance, when an employee converts to part-time status and coverage is not offered to such part-time employees; when a part-time employee does not work the requisite hours in a pay period to be covered; or when the employee does not pay the applicable portion of the premium required for coverage.

QUALIFICATIONS OF THE PROVIDER

Health plan contracts generally require that a hospital provider be appropriately licensed and certified by the Medicare program to render hospital services to that program. The contract also may require that the hospital be accredited by the Joint Commission on Accreditation of Healthcare Organizations (JCAHO).

Health plan contracts generally require that a physician provider be appropriately licensed in the state to practice medicine, and also may require that the physician be eligible to participate in the Medicare program. In addition, the physician may have to be appropriately credentialed in accordance with the health plan's credentialing process.

SERVICES TO BE PROVIDED

The contract also should set forth the services which will be provided and their availability. Typically, a hospital only would want to commit to provide those services which it has available on its premises. It would not want to be required to provide physician services unless those physicians were employed by the hospital or under contract to provide such services, such as hospital-based physicians. Even where a hospital has hospital-based physicians, however, it may be preferable to have the health plan contract directly with them to minimize negotiations with the physicians.

Often the health plan contract includes a schedule of the services which the hospital will provide. Occasionally, the hospital merely agrees to provide those services which are available on its campus. The health plans also require that the services of the hospital are offered to health plan patients on the same basis as to non–health plan patients. Similar provisions are placed in the physicians' contracts with the health plans. In a capitated arrangement, it is particularly important to define which individuals are entitled to the services.

Physicians at least will contract to provide the services which they can offer. In a capitated arrangement, however, both hospitals and physicians typically might provide a broader range of services, *e.g.*, all hospital or all physician services, with the expectation that they will subcontract for the services which they cannot provide. When hospitals or physicians contractually commit themselves to provide more services than they can provide on their own, such providers must ensure that they have contracted with other providers, so that all the services which they have agreed with the health plan to provide will be provided in a quality, cost-effective manner. In addition, the providers need to ensure that the health plan will not object to such subcontracting. Furthermore, whether preexisting conditions are covered and whether out-of-area services are covered are important considerations under capitation.

COMPENSATION

The compensation set forth in a contract should be clearly identified. As noted in Chapter 3, compensation arrangements may take many different forms from discounts from charges, per diems for hospitals, fee schedules, case rates, DRGs, package or global pricing to capitation. Health plans seek to compensate providers only for covered services which are medically necessary.

Time for Payment

The time for payment of such compensation should be set forth in the contract. If a provider is being paid on a capitated basis, the contract may provide that the provider should receive its capitation check on a date near the beginning of the month. If the provider is being paid only after the submission of bills or statements for services rendered, the contract should delineate the nature of the bill which the providers should submit, *e.g.*, on a UB 92 form or whatever other form may be required. In addition, the contract should state by what date a provider must submit a bill after a service is rendered or if it can submit a bill during the service (in the case of a lengthy stay), and by what date the health plan is required to pay the provider after the receipt of the bill.

Often, the contract provides that the health plan is only required to pay the provider after the receipt of a "clean claim." That is, a claim which includes the proper billing information and related forms and has the correct information. The definition of "clean claim," however, should not be so restrictive as to make it too difficult for providers to be paid for legitimate claims. Some contracts provide that claims may be submitted electronically. An explanation of such submissions should be part of the contract.

If part of a claim is disputed, some health plan contracts provide that the health plan should pay the nondisputed portion of the bill and let the remainder of the bill proceed through a dispute resolution process. Such a provision is particularly important for a provider where the bill is substantial, and/or for a lengthy stay.

Interest or Reversion to Charges

Providers often seek to include provisions in payor contracts which provide for the payment of interest or the reversion of the contract rates to billed charges if a health plan does not pay within a certain period of time. Health plans generally do not object to placing timely payment provisions in their contracts, but they are reluctant to agree to pay interest or have the contract revert to charges in the event of late payment. If a contract provides for interest, the contract should delineate the rate and how it is calculated. The parties to such agreements should pay particular attention to any usury laws which govern the maximum rate of interest payable.

Although few contracts may provide that if a health plan does not pay a provider in a timely manner for the services rendered the bill will revert to billed charges, there may be justification in some instances for such a provision. For example, if the provider is giving the discount for prompt payment and there is not prompt payment, the provider has not received the benefit of its bargain. However, the health plan likely will argue that its bargain was to pay the discounted rates, and at most the provider has a time value of money argument.

UTILIZATION REVIEW AND MANAGEMENT AND QUALITY ASSURANCE

Health plans typically have utilization review, and management and quality assurance plans, incorporated into their operations. They expect that providers will adhere to and cooperate with such programs. Utilization review and management plans permit the health plans to review and manage the utilization of the services of the hospital, physicians, and other providers and suppliers. Nurses and physicians are used in this process to ensure the cost-effective delivery of quality care.

In a quality assurance plan, the health plan seeks to ensure that its beneficiaries are receiving high-quality care. The care rendered by the hospitals, physicians, and other providers and suppliers is reviewed and quality improvement mechanisms may be employed. The utilization review and management and quality assurance plans should be appended to the managed care contract or incorporated by reference. The hospital and physicians should have actual copies of the plan, not merely descriptions of them. Any modifications to such plans should be disseminated to the providers in ample time for them to implement the effects of such plans. In addition, any material modifications or revisions which could have a financial effect on a provider should be subject to the approval and consent of the provider prior to implementation. Occasionally, particularly in capitated arrangements, these functions might be delegated to the providers. If they are delegated, the providers will undoubtedly want to obtain higher capitation payments than if the duties were not delegated, because the providers will be doing more for the capitation payments.

The health plans, on the other hand, will want to maintain flexible utilization review and management and quality assurance plans and continually update them to ensure that they facilitate the cost-effective delivery of quality care. They will not want to seek the consent of the providers in their networks for any changes to such plans because they view such plans to be within their purview, and seeking the agreement of all the providers in the provider network could be a very lengthy process.

However, there might be revisions to utilization review and management and quality assurance plans which carry a substantial cost to a provider. For example, if the health plan starts delegating some portion of these plans to a provider, there is a cost to the provider of assuming that function. If the provider is not appropriately compensated for doing so, its agreement with the health plan could be materially affected.

PRIOR AUTHORIZATION, CONCURRENT REVIEW, AND RETROSPECTIVE REVIEW

Typically, a managed care contract addresses such issues as prior authorization, concurrent review, retrospective review, and the consequences of such reviews. These provisions are most important when providers are not paid on a capitated basis. Where they are paid on a capitated basis, the providers might assume these functions because the decision to render treatment is a cost to the provider, not the subject of an additional payment.

Prior Authorization

Prior authorization is the process by which a provider is required to obtain from the health plan prior authorization to treat a beneficiary. The provider would want to be assured that it understands the prior authorization procedures, and that they are workable for the institution and the physicians. A provider also would want to be able to rely on a health plan's prior authorization, unless, of course, the information provided to the health plan was incorrect. That is, a provider would not want a health plan to be able to argue later that its prior authorization was ineffective, absent some extenuating circumstances. The health plan, on the other hand, would not want to be obligated to pay a provider for healthcare services if the health plan would not have authorized the care had it known all the facts.

Concurrent Review

Many health plans conduct concurrent review of a patient's stay. During that review, a health plan may authorize a continued stay in a hospital and/or assist in making arrangements to discharge or transfer a patient. By actively being involved in the review and management of a patient's care and stay in the hospital, the health plan can help ensure that the most cost-effective care is delivered to the patient, and that an inpatient is discharged at the earliest possible date. However, physicians often believe that such involvement in the process adversely effects the physician's ability to manage care. Such concerns are less prevalent today than years ago, when health plans started managing more of a patient's care.

Retrospective Review

Health plans conduct a retrospective review to review a patient's admission, stay, or course of treatment after it has occurred. Providers want to be assured that, should retrospective reviews occur, they will not result in retroactive denial of payment. Health plans do not want to pay for hospital stays or treatment which they do not believe are covered. It may come to the health plan's attention through retrospective review, once the patient has been discharged, that the patient did not need to be admitted to the hospital, the patient could have been discharged earlier, or the patient received services which were not necessary or were not in the appropriate setting. A health plan would want to be assured that it is not required to pay a provider for such services. On the other hand, a provider which has been subjected to preauthorization and continuous stay review would argue that it should not be denied any payment because the health plan had the opportunity to deny the admission prior to its incurrence or to suggest that the patient be discharged earlier through continued stay review.

A health plan, however, may be able to make a retrospective determination as to whether an emergency admission was a "true" emergency warranting admission to the hospital. In making such a determination, the health plan likely will rely on the definition of emergency in the health plan contract. As a result, as mentioned above, it is important for providers to ensure that definition of emergency is consistent with the practices of the hospital and the physicians in attendance.

RISK POOLS

Increasingly, health plan contracts contain risk pools, but particularly when the providers receive capitation payments. Risk pools are a means of risk sharing. The terms and conditions of any risk pools should be specifically delineated in the contract. Are the risk pools shared between the provider and the health plan for low utilization? Are they shared among providers? How are they administered? Does the provider have both an upside and a downside risk?

It is necessary to delineate who is at risk, for what, and is there a fund to stabilize that risk. For example, the risk pool might be tied to hospital utilization in days per thousand enrollees. If a specific target is not met because utilization is too high, both the physicians and the hospital may be adversely effected because of a decrease in the monies available for distribution. If utilization is below the target or budget, the hospital and physicians might share in the additional monies remaining in the risk pool. Furthermore, a risk stabilization fund may be employed which might stabilize the providers' risk of adverse utilization over a certain period of time. A risk pool may also be established as a contingency fund for IBNRs or other payments.

TERM

The term of a managed care contract should be set forth unambiguously. Often, managed care companies will want the hospital or physician to enter into a contract which is automatically renewable on a year-to-year basis to ensure that it has continued provider coverage for its beneficiaries. Such contracts are often called "evergreen contracts." The problem with such agreements, however, from the perspective of the provider, is that the provider is undoubtedly participating in numerous contracts and that it might miss the date for termination. Unless there is a short without cause termination, the contract will automatically renew at the last year's rates. Although an early termination provision may reduce somewhat these concerns on the part of the providers, a health plan may want to ensure that it has time to replace part of its provider network if providers tender an early termination notice. Inasmuch as providers typically want to renegotiate higher rates each year, if they miss the date for renegotiation, it might be difficult to renegotiate retroactive rates. Of course, a provider should seek to renegotiate new payment rates, which are retroactive to the anniversary date, on a yearly basis. A health plan will want any new rates effective only on the later of the anniversary date or on the date on which the rates were agreed upon by the parties.

TERMINATION

There are generally two types of termination provisions in health plan contracts. There are provisions which provide for the termination by either party without cause or termination with cause. Without cause termination provisions are typically 30-, 60-, 90-, 120-, or 180-day provisions. With cause termination provisions often involve elaborate issues with respect to material breaches and notice and cure periods. That is, a party may be required to state the basis upon which it believes there is a breach of contract by the other party and provide the other party with an opportunity to cure that breach of contract. If the second party cures the breach, the contract remains in force and effect. If it does not, the contract terminates. Obviously, if there is a without cause termination provision, the parties are more likely to utilize that provision than a with cause termination provision. And with the latter, of course, there is less room for dispute.

Providers should be particularly careful to ensure that notice and cure provisions do not apply to the payment provisions. That is, if a health plan has agreed to pay a provider within 30 days, a provider might want to terminate the agreement for breach of contract. If the agreement includes a 30-day notice and a 30-day cure provision whereby the provider has to give the health plan 30 days notice of its intent to terminate the agreement, and the health plan has 30 days to cure or pay, the health plan actually has 90 days, not 30, to pay.

Health plan contracts generally afford a health plan the ability to terminate the contract immediately if the safety of the patients is in jeopardy, the physician's license is lost or suspended, the physician is convicted of a felony, is incapacitated, or is excluded from the Medicare and Medicaid programs. With respect to a hospital provider, if the hospital loses its license to operate a hospital, its Medicare certification, or JCAHO accreditation, or is excluded from the Medicare and Medicaid programs, a health plan generally is able to immediately terminate the health plan contract.

INSURANCE

Managed care plans often require that healthcare providers, whether hospitals or physicians, maintain insurance which would cover them for general and professional liability and for their performance under the agreement. The amount of insurance coverage may be negotiable, but providers will want to maintain adequate insurance coverage for their actions and operations in any event. Often, the health plans seek to obtain copies of certificates of insurance evidencing the insurance coverage of the providers and negotiate for notice of cancellation of such coverage prior to its effective date. Some plans also may request that the health plan be listed on the provider's policy as an additional named insured to ensure that the health plan is covered and will have notice of any such termination. Of course, a provider would prefer not to agree to such latter requirement. If a provider has a "claims made" policy, the health plan may request assurance that the "tail" coverage will be available to the provider by the insurer, and that the provider will purchase such tail coverage.

Providers also should ensure that the health plan maintains the necessary coverage for its potential liabilities under the contract, including its utilization review decisions. However, it should be noted that many health plans are insurance companies, and they suggest that they should not have to insure for such utilization review activities. Even if they are not insurers, they seek to limit their liability for such decisions. One such means of attempting to limit the health plan's liability in this regard is by including independent contractor provisions in their contracts which are in part meant to insulate a health plan from the decisions of a provider with respect to treatment.

INDEPENDENT CONTRACTORS

Many health plan contracts include provisions which state that the parties are not acting on behalf of each other or as their agents, but they are independent contractors. A health plan would be interested in including such language to suggest that all decisions with respect to treatment are ultimately those of the physician and the hospital, suggesting that all attendant liabilities should lie with the physician or the hospital. The health plans take the position that they only make coverage and payment decisions. Obviously, a provider does not want a health plan to be its agent in the delivery of healthcare services, but a provider would want a health plan to be responsible for its utilization review decisions.

INDEMNITY AND/OR HOLD HARMLESS

Occasionally, contracts include indemnity and/or hold harmless provisions which provide that one party will indemnify and/or hold harmless the other party in the event that the first party's actions result in liability to the second party. In such instances, the provider should at least ensure that such provisions are mutual and are acceptable to its insurance carriers. Liabilities incurred as a result of indemnity and hold harmless provisions often are not covered by insurance because they are viewed as contractual obligations.

APPEALS MECHANISMS

The provider wants to ensure mechanisms that provide for timely appeals are included in the contract, and that if the individual or entity which ultimately decides whether payment made is the health plan, that there is some further means to appeal, *e.g.*, bringing the matter to arbitration or resorting to the courts. If a patient is in need of a particular procedure or in the hospital needing additional treatment or a longer stay, it is necessary to have a quick appeals process which accommodates decisions in the context of the applicable time-frame needed for treatment. Although the appeals procedure might proceed through a number of levels, it is important that early in the process that some professional with experience in treatment of the type required by the patient be available for consultation, if necessary. The provider and the beneficiary should be able to make their case to the health plan and have some level of further appeal within the health plan. Final appeals might be heard in an arbitration proceeding or proceed to court.

DISPUTE RESOLUTION

An appeals mechanism in the contract which establishes the provider's right of appeal of utilization review or coverage decisions by the health plan may be different from a dispute resolution provision in the managed care contract. Such a utilization review dispute resolution section may provide that utilization review and coverage decisions must first proceed through the appeals mechanism prior to proceeding through dispute resolution. Other disputes may be subject to the standard dispute resolution procedures in the managed care contract. Such provisions may require that the parties first employ nonbinding mediation. It may provide for binding arbitration pursuant to certain procedures, or it may provide that any disputes should proceed directly to court.

The nature of any such arbitration proceeding should be set forth in the contract, including the number of arbitrators, how they are chosen, and the necessary experience or skills they should have. In addition, the nature of the arbitration procedure and the rules governing it can be set forth. If a matter will proceed to litigation in the courts, the contract could provide the agreed upon venue for such court and the choice of laws.

GRIEVANCE PROCEDURES

Many health plans include grievance procedures, or require that the provider present a grievance procedure subject to approval by the health plan prior to implementation. A grievance procedure should afford the beneficiary the opportunity to air a grievance and obtain a response from the provider about its possible resolution. Occasionally, the health plan will want to be made aware of any grievances submitted by an enrollee. Many hospitals and physicians have patient satisfaction surveys. Providers will want to be careful that such survey responses are not treated as grievances.

INSOLVENCY

It may be important for providers to establish some protection against the insolvency of the payor in the health plan contract. An often used means to obtain this protection is a section which provides that, in the event of bankruptcy of a health plan, the provider is no longer required to provide services to the health plan's beneficiaries. Generally, however, a bankruptcy court will not uphold such a provision because a bankruptcy proceeding stays the *status quo*, which is that the provider has agreed to render services to a health plan's beneficiaries. In a bankruptcy proceeding, the health plan may decide whether it wants to accept or reject the preexisting contract.

As a result, providers often attempt to include language in health plan contracts to enable the provider to terminate the agreement prior to bankruptcy at early warning signs of a plan's financial problems. Such provisions might include a requirement that the plan forward to the provider copies of its audited and unaudited financial statements. They might allow the provider to terminate the contract early for late payment if the health plan becomes in arrears by a certain amount; or require periodic payments, sometimes known as current financing, by the health plan to the provider to ensure that the health plan is always current. In the case of providers doing a substantial amount of business with a health plan, the provider may request a letter of credit.

In a capitated arrangement, a health plan will want to be assured that the provider does not become insolvent, particularly if the provider is responsible for paying claims of other providers from the monies which the capitated provider received. Health plans may require financial statements of such providers, assurances of their ability to perform, or even letters of credit.

ASSIGNMENT

It may be preferable to include a prohibition against assignment in health plan contracts, extending both to the benefit of the provider and the health plan. A health plan or provider might want to be able to assign a health plan contract to a related organization, but the nature of that related organization may not be the same as the organization originally entering into the contract. In addition, in most of these contracts, the health plan has chosen the hospitals and physicians with which it desires to contract, and it would not want the providers to assign the contract to another hospital or physician group without the health plan's consent. The providers have bargained for a contract with a particular plan; they would not necessarily want the health plan assigning their contract to a shell or thinly capitalized entity even if it was related to the health plan.

Occasionally, however, health plan contracts permit the health plan or provider to assign the contract to an entity which is part of a corporate reorganization, or if at least 50% ownership in the entity remains the same. A health plan wants to be careful because owner-ship of the medical group or hospital may change. If such a transac-tion is accomplished by the sale of stock, the antiassignment provi-sions may not be triggered. Where the parties are required to obtain the consent of the other party, a clause might be inserted which provides that such consent will not be unreasonably withheld. Such a provision gives the parties assurances that the other party will not reject an assignment based on a whim, but that an assignment will not be automatic, particularly if there is a justifiable reason for the other party objecting to it.

PROPRIETARY RIGHTS AND ADVERTISING

Health plan contracts often include provisions which permit the parties to maintain their rights over their proprietary symbols, names, information, and so on. Although the contract may give each party the ability to use the other parties' name in advertising or promotion, there are often limitations on such advertising, market-ing, or publicity. For example, an advertisement featuring only the provider and the health plan may have to be approved by the party not seeking to conduct the advertising. Of course, the mere inclusion of a provider's name in the health plan's provider booklet should not require prior permission. In fact, generally that is what the provider bargains for—having its name placed in the health plan's roster of providers to facilitate the choice of that provider by an enrollee or beneficiary. It is helpful to include in the agreement that any prior permission with respect to use of names, symbols, *etc.*, will be revoked upon termination of the agreement. However, a health plan only should be required to amend or revise its provider booklet or direc-tory at its usual and customary date for doing so, which should not exceed six months to one year. In addition, where a health plan forwards updates to its beneficiaries, a provider wants to ensure that such updates note that the provider is no longer a member of that provider network.

BILLING THE BENEFICIARY

HMO contracts generally must include a provision stating that the provider will not bill the patient for any services unless the provider is authorized to do so by the health plan, *e.g.*, for copayments or noncovered services for which the patient has contractually agreed to pay prior to the provider rendering the services. Such provisions are required by federal and state laws governing HMOs. Increasingly, however, non-HMO health plans include such language in their agreements, although there may be no statutory requirement for them to do so. Obviously, in a non-HMO contract, a provider would want the flexibility to collect from the patient if the health plan did not pay for the services rendered. Of course, a provider attempting to collect from patients in this manner would not foster good relations between the health plan and its beneficiaries. As a result, non-HMO plans often attempt to include provisions in their agreements which preclude a provider from billing a patent unless the patient has been advised in writing by a provider of its responsibility to pay and the patient has executed such a document evidencing his or her agreement.

ACCESS TO RECORDS

Health plans generally require access to patient and provider records as part of their agreements with providers. Providers want to exclude from review all records which might be subject to certain confidentiality protections granted by state law, such as peer review records, and often any other records which they do not want to make available to the health plan. Applicable state law, however, may grant access to certain records to health plans consistent with patient confidentiality.

Although a provider might not be concerned with whether a health plan reviews certain medical records of its beneficiaries, the provider will want to ensure that the health plan maintains any necessary confidentiality and obtains the permission of the patient, either through some written consent or statutory authorization, to review the record. The provider will want to ensure that the health plan only has access to the records of its beneficiaries and upon reasonable written notice, *e.g.*, three business days or 72 hours, not including weekends and holidays.

Access to other provider records, such as billing and financial records, should be limited to those records necessary for review of a patient stay. Such records might include the detailed billing information associated with a patient stay and backup information for services provided, such as charge tickets. A health plan should not have unlimited access to all provider records because of the burdensome nature of such access.

Similarly, a provider should not have unlimited access to a health plan's financial records. Access to records of a health plan to ensure its financial visibility and stability should be sufficient. However, if either party has information to believe that the other party may be in financial distress or insolvent, that party should be able to request copies of financial records which would support or refute this understanding, to ensure the provider a reasonable expectation of being paid by the health plan, or that the health plan will continue to have a viable provider network.

COST OF RECORD RETRIEVAL, AUDIT, AND PHOTOCOPIES

Providers often seek to charge a health plan for the providers' cost of record retrieval, audit, and photocopies. The providers' charges, if any, should be reasonable and should be set forth in its agreement with the health plan. What is reasonable to a provider, however, is not necessarily reasonable to a health plan. If the agreement provides that the health plan will pay the providers' costs for such activities, the health plan will likely interpret those costs to be variable costs, and the hospital will interpret the costs to be fully allocated costs. It is best to be as specific as possible to reduce any possibility of disagreement at a later date.

COORDINATION OF BENEFITS

A health plan contract should include a coordination of benefits provision to establish that benefits are to be coordinated according to applicable state law or in a particular manner set forth in the agreement. Such a provision should state who is entitled to coordinate benefits, which is particularly important in capitated arrangements. If the health plan is the primary payor, a provider will want to ensure that it will pay in full subject to the terms of the contract. If the health plan is secondary, the provider will want to ensure that the health plan will pay the difference between the provider's charges and the amount paid for by the other health plan and the beneficiary. Often, health plans will want the contract to provide that if the health plan is secondary, it will pay the difference between what the primary health plan paid and what the secondary health plan would have paid if it had been primary. As a result, the secondary health plan is generally required to pay very little, if anything, to the provider.

Providers should know that, occasionally, a health plan which is secondary contends that there is no amount left for them to pay when a health plan which is primary has paid the provider, because the provider has agreed to accept the payment from the primary health plan as payment in full. Careful drafting of all the providers' health plan contracts is necessary to reduce the possibility of such an argument being successful.

COLLECTION OF DEDUCTIBLES AND COPAYMENTS

Health plan contracts might include provisions setting forth the applicable deductibles and copayments for which a patient is responsible. The agreement might provide that it is the responsibility of the providers to collect these amounts. It may even specifically preclude the provider from waiving any such amounts. Even if the contract does not specifically preclude the waiver of deductibles and copayments, health plans often take the position that providers are precluded from doing so because such monies result in a reduction in the provider's charges which is inappropriately not passed on to the health plan, and the provider has frustrated the health plan's ability to contain its costs through appropriate utilization.

CONFIDENTIALITY

Many health plan contracts include a clarifying clause which provides that the contract terms, particularly the price terms, shall remain confidential, subject to applicable law and regulation. Thus, if a state or federal agency was statutorily authorized to review all or part of the contract, there would be no breach of its terms.

EXCLUSIVITY AND INCENTIVES

Many providers want to negotiate exclusivity provisions in health plan agreements or ensure that incentives exist for the beneficiary to use the providers. If a provider has offered a health plan a discount, it generally expects some additional value for that discount whether in terms of patients or lives. One way to ensure this is for the provider to have an exclusive contract with the health plan for a particular area. Another less effective way is for the health plan to limit the number of contracting or preferred providers and for the health plan to ensure that there are incentives for the beneficiaries to visit a contracting or preferred provider. Such incentives might include lower copayments or lower deductibles for the beneficiaries who visit contracting preferred providers. Such provisions also should be set forth in the applicable benefit plans.

MOST-FAVORED NATIONS CLAUSES

A contracting health plan may require that a provider extend to it the lowest discount it offers to any health plan. Such a provision often is referred to as a "most-favored nations" clause. Obviously, a provider would not want to enter into such an agreement because the provider's contract is merely at the lowest level of any contract it enters into. Although it may not necessarily be viewed as illegal, if either the health plan or the provider has considerable market dominance, such an agreement might be seen as restraint of trade and in violation of the antitrust laws.

CATHOLIC CLAUSE

If a provider is a catholic facility or individual, the health plan contract might exempt the provider from any services which are inconsistent with certain ethical directives. Thus the Catholic facility or individual would not be required to provide abortions or elective sterilizations.

NONDISCRIMINATION

Health plan contracts generally provide that the providers cannot discriminate against beneficiaries based on race, ethnic origin, age, sex, disability, or sexual orientation. These nondiscrimination provisions help ensure that all health plan beneficiaries will receive appropriate treatment.

BOILERPLATE

Health plan contracts also typically include the following types of boilerplate provisions, including authority, notices, force majeure, severability, counterparts, governing law, etc.

Authority

The parties should warrant or agree that they have the requisite authority to enter into the managed care contract.

Notices

There should be a provision in the agreement which states to whom and where notices under the agreement should be sent, the manner in which notice must be made, and when they are effective. For example, should notice be provided by certified mail, return receipt requested? May it be given through an expedited mail service, hand delivery, or so on? In addition, when will such notice be effective—upon receipt, two days after mailing, *etc.*?

Force Majeure

Managed care contracts often include *force majeure* clauses which provide that in the event of an act of God, such as an earthquake, hurricane, tornado, fire, or some event which is not within the control of the providers, such as a strike or work stoppage, performance under the agreement might be suspended for some period of time. However, in a capitated arrangement, providers are more likely to continue to have the obligation to arrange the necessary care for their enrollees, even if they do not have to provide the services directly.

Severability and Counterparts

Severability provisions provide that if one provision in the contract is held to be invalid, the remainder of the contract will be upheld. A counterparts provision permits the parties to sign on different pages; and the combination of those signatures will be valid for an executed contract.

Governing Law

A governing law provision sets forth the state law which will apply to interpretations under the contract.

CONCLUSION

Managed care contract terms are numerous, and they can be complex and confusing. It is important to understand the nature of these contracts and their complexities. In addition, any ambiguities should be minimized as much as possible. Failure to do so can result in a substantial financial loss for a party.

6

The Importance of the Managed Care Relationship, Who Receives Payment, and Who Accepts Risk

As relationships moved from the indemnity arena—where an insurer paid a physician or hospital based on an assignment of benefits—to managed care relationships—where a health plan pays the physician or hospital based on a direct relationship—it became necessary to memorialize these relationships with a written contract. Although Chapter 5 discusses the nature of these contracts, this chapter discusses the importance of the managed care relationship, whom the health plans pay and for what, and who can accept risk.

RELATIONSHIPS BETWEEN HEALTH PLANS AND PHYSICIANS

Individual Physicians and Physician Groups

When health plans first began to formalize their relationships with providers through managed care contracts, the contract generally was with the provider providing the service, which might be the individual physician, physician group, or hospital. Where a health plan does not pay physicians on a capitated basis, individual physicians may be able to retain relationships with health plans for some period of time. However, as health plans increasingly capitate physicians, contracting with physician groups, in lieu of individual physicians, becomes more important. Where such groups contract with managed care plans, there can be an increased number of lives for which they are responsible which will reduce the overall risk of the group, compared to an individual physician.

As managed care plans merge and consolidate their operations, and as more patients are covered by such plans, it is of paramount important for such providers to have good relationships with the managed care plans. Many physicians in some parts of the country which are now dominated by managed care did not enter into relationships with managed care companies in earlier years, and they are now finding that their failure to do so has closed them out of the ability to treat significant patient populations. Similarly, many physicians who have failed to align with medical groups are experiencing a similar fate.

Many PPOs wanted as broad of a network as possible to enable them to more effectively market to prospective employers a wide choice of providers. PPOs typically paid the individual physician; the physician group, if it was integrated; or, if the group was an IPA, either the individual physicians or the IPA. HMOs, however, were more likely to limit their provider network because of their ability to better manage care in a more restrictive network, and for those HMOs paying providers on a capitation basis, it was necessary to limit provider networks to assure that the providers in the network had enough managed care lives to make participation in the network worthwhile and to reduce their risk.

(PPOs and other health plans increasingly sought to enter contracts with physician groups for physician services because it significantly decreased their cost and time associated with managed care contracting. For example, a single contract with a group of 17 physicians eliminates the need for 17 individual contracts.)

Many HMOs paid individual physicians on a fee schedule basis, but increasingly, the HMOs sought to contract with physician groups on a risk basis. Risk pools were employed where physicians might be paid on a fee schedule or modified fee-for-service basis with a withhold. The total compensation to the physicians might be subject to a cap which was determined based on capitated payments per member per month. If the physicians kept utilization down, they could keep all or part of the money remaining in the risk pool. They might only keep part because the health plan was helping to manage the system and administering the risk pool, and as a result, it might share in it. Physicians, increasingly, began to receive full risk capitation payments from health plans where the physicians managed the system. It became increasingly important to health plans that physicians be organized in groups which could manage care.

Physician groups soon began to realize the value of their contractual relationships with the health plans—relationships which were particularly valuable if they were exclusive or limited in nature. As health plans matured as entities, they began to realize that there was much value in a stable base of providers, and they became reluctant to upset that stable base unless they could not negotiate acceptable price terms. In addition, health plans grew more reluctant about permitting new providers to become part of their networks because of the negative reaction to their doing so by the existing providers and their fear of having to grant greater rate increases to their existing providers.

In less mature markets, enterprising physician groups who watched the developments in managed care in the more mature markets sought to obtain exclusive relationships with health plans to ensure their ability to continue to serve patients and to be dominant players in a market. In fact, such physicians recognized that such relationships might be at the core of their success.

The Effect of the Expansion of Physician Networks

Physicians realizing the importance of managed care contracts also have realized the importance of growing their individual groups or networks in a manner which affords them the ability to control more patients or lives. For example, a small, primary care medical group which has a contract with a health plan might add to its capacity in a number of ways. It could take on additional shareholders or partners or employ additional physicians. The strategy works best when the physician group's practice has developed to such an extent that the growth in the practice necessitates the addition of physicians. Where such physicians are added to the practice in this manner, the managed care plan might merely add more physicians to the managed care contract, or if that is not necessary, to the roster of individual providers making up the medical group. The physicians, of course, will need to be properly credentialed by the health plan's credentialing procedures.

Another means by which a medical group can expand is by contracting with other physicians or physician groups on an independent contractor basis to provide services through the first medical group. Many medical groups often have obtained additional capacity through independent contractor relationships with physicians as an alternative to employing them. Such relationships afford greater flexibility to the medical group, which might not be able to ensure that there will be enough business for a new physician shareholder or employee.

Medical groups also have contracted with other medical groups to provide services. Originally, such relationships may have started because a primary care group wanted to offer an additional physician service on its site, *e.g.*, cardiology. The primary care medical group might have contracted with the cardiology medical group for a cardiologist to practice one half day a week at the primary care group's site, and the services might have been provided through the primary care medical group.

Newer relationships have emerged, however, because of a recognition of the value of a managed care contract with a health plan. For example, an individual physician or physician group that wants to access a managed care contract might attempt to contract through a medical group that has an existing contract with a health plan. Mere willingness of the medical group contracting with the health plan to do so, however, is not sufficient to extend the contract to the second medical group. The health plan will generally consider a number of issues in deciding whether to do so. Does it need the additional capacity or coverage in a particular geographic area? Will the addition of the medical group adversely affect its relationship with another medical group? Can this medical group manage care?

The first medical group might be willing (or even anxious) to add a second medical group if it affords the first medical group the ability to expand its overall network and increase the number of patients or lives it controls, assuming the contract with the health plan remains with the first medical group and the second medical group is merely a contractor through the first.

The Effect of Acquisitions, Mergers, and Consolidations of Medical Groups

Another method of expansion for medical groups is the acquisition of other medical groups, mergers, or consolidations. With the acquisition of another medical group, the members of the acquired medical group become members of the acquiring medical group. The health plans likely will treat such an arrangement as more significant than adding one or two new physicians. The issues for the health plan, however, can be complicated depending upon other provider relationships.

With a merger of medical groups, the contracts are likely to remain with the group into which the other group merged. In a merger one entity merges into the surviving entity. Consolidations present a more interesting case because both entities disappear into a new entity. The new entity as a result will not have had the managed care contract.

HOSPITALS, ANCILLARY PROVIDERS, AND INTEGRATED DELIVERY SYSTEMS

Hospital and ancillary providers receive payment from the health plans for their respective services. Although hospitals often seek to contract with health plans for physician services, ancillary providers generally only seek to contract for their own services.

Physician Hospital Organizations (PHOs), Management Services Organizations (MSOs), medical foundations, and fully integrated delivery systems may be limited in their ability to accept payments from health plans by applicable state law and may even be subject to licensure requirements. In such an event, the entities comprising the delivery system may have to contract with the payors and assign their revenues to the PHO, MSO, medical foundation, or other entity in the integrated delivery system. If such entities are not limited by state law in contracting for hospital, physicians, and ancillary services, there will be more inherent flexibility in the integrated delivery system.

THE IMPORTANCE OF THE MANAGED CARE CONTRACT

Those medical groups which have contracts with health plans can significantly control the flow of patients. Thus, a small medical group which can add to its capacity and network by subcontracts can control a substantial number of lives and patients. If a subcontracting medical group or physician in that medical group becomes unhappy with the first medical group and leaves the network, it leaves with no managed care contracts unless it retained some when it joined the network. The prognosis for developing a private medical practice in many areas of the county is not good for a new physician or a physician new to the area. Such a physician would likely seek affiliation with another medical group, employment by a health plan, hospital or other entity, or another relationship which assured patient access.

Physicians contracting for other physicians' services with health plans may not seem unusual because even if a primary care physician contracts for all physician services, including those of a specialist, both physicians practice medicine. Physicians, however, are now seeking to contract for hospital services. Recognizing that a very large portion of the healthcare dollar is expended on hospital services, physicians often desire to contract with health plans for hospital services. Of course, if the physicians own a hospital, there would be no problem with the entity which owns that hospital directly contracting with a health plan. If the physicians do not, it may be difficult for them to contract for hospital services.

WHOM HEALTH PLANS PAY, AND FOR WHAT

Physicians for Hospital Services

One must look to state law to determine whether a health plan may pay physicians for hospital services on a capitated basis where the physicians do not own a hospital, but merely intend to subcontract for such services with a hospital. For instance, a provider contracting with another provider for a service which the first provider cannot provide directly is seen as incurring an insurance risk, and such assumption of risk or acting like an insurance company or health plan may be regulated by state law.

If physicians are able to subcontract for hospital services where they do not own a hospital and that hospital has Medicare and Medicaid patients who have been referred to the hospital by those physicians, a Medicare fraud and abuse issue could arise. If the physicians retain a portion of the payment from the health plan to the physicians for the hospital care, it might be argued that the physicians are retaining an amount for their referral of Medicare and Medicaid patients to the hospital. Physicians would want to ensure that their referrals of Medicare and Medicaid patients was not influenced by their contract with the hospitals for capitated patients. In any event, in many situations, the possibility of physicians contracting for hospital services where they do not own a hospital is moot because a health plan may not desire to contract with a physician group for hospital services. This issue is becoming increasingly important, and some physicians are most interested in contracting for both physician and hospital services. Where not prohibited by state law, such arrangements are likely to grow in acceptance.

Hospitals for Physician Services

Hospitals often contract for physician services with health plans. Hospitals are particularly interested in being able to contract on behalf of physicians to enable the hospital to be able to control the capitated dollars and thus the revenue flow into the system. In fact when a hospital is treated as a cost center, as under a capitated system, its ability to survive may be based on its ability to control part of the revenue flow.

Many hospitals may contract primarily for the services of hospital-based physicians, but may include the services of employed or contracted physicians. However, in states which have prohibitions against the corporate practice of medicine or restrictive medical practice acts, the services of hospital-based physicians are likely to be the only ones for which the health plan will contract with the hospital, and even such a relationship may be on an agency basis. The regulatory issues and their interpretations by hospitals, hospital associations, physicians, medical societies, and states are often not clear.

Physicians or Hospital for Ancillary Services

Health plans typically will pay either physicians or hospitals for ancillary services, such as laboratory or radiology services, if those services might be provided by physicians or hospitals or if the physicians or hospitals own such ancillary services. However, more restrictive state laws addressing the assumption of such risk for ancillary services may require that the party assuming such risk be licensed for and own such ancillary services, not merely be in a position to contract for them.

RESTRICTIONS ON A HEALTH PLAN'S ABILITY TO PAY PROVIDERS

State Fee-Splitting Restrictions

In many states, absent an integrated medical group, there are restrictions on paying modified fee-for-service payments to providers who do not render the services for which they are paid because of state law prohibitions on fee splitting. As payment systems move to capitation, providers seek capitation and look toward controlling those capitation payments; such state fee-splitting restrictions are likely to be less of an issue, but some might arguably apply to certain capitation arrangements.

State Restrictions on Taking Risk

Various states have laws which prohibit or limit the ability of providers to take risk. Others seem not to address the situation or to understand it in the context of managed care contracting under capitation. A physician group which is paid on a capitated basis, a fixed amount pmpm for physician services, is at risk for the provision of physician services to the patient population. Generally, it is thought that a provider may be at risk for the services it can provide. However, the provider may be precluded by state law from assuming risk for services it cannot provide. Where such is the case, the analysis may be clear with respect to hospital services: if the physician group does not own a hospital, it would not be able to assume the risk for the provision of hospital services. However, the case is less clear with respect to a primary care physician group assuming the risk for all physician services where the primary care group cannot directly provide the specialty physician services with physicians in its group.

The better reasoned analysis is to permit such primary care physicians to assume the risk for all physician services because physician groups have contracted with other physicians to provide services through other groups for years and, more importantly, such assumption of risk makes it easier for the primary care medical group to manage care. It should be noted that where the primary care group subcapitates another physician or medical group, that subcapitated medical group also has assumed risk, and that assumption of risk must be analyzed under applicable state statutes.

Physicians often seek to be capitated for certain ancillary services. The following questions might arise as to whether a physician group might be capitated for such services. Do the physicians own such ancillary services? Are they licensed to provide such services? Could they be licensed to provide such services? If they own such ancillaries, there should be no problem with any health plan capitating the physicians for such services. The situation is less clear if the physicians merely are licensed to provide such services. Distinctions might be made on the basis of whether the physician group could operate a laboratory in its office or a pharmacy, whereas operating a hospital might create different issues.

CONCLUSION

As noted above, the managed care relationship is becoming increasingly important, and the focus is on who has that direct relationship. It is important to ascertain whom health plans pay, and for what, and who can accept risk.

7

The Development of Organizational Structures to Manage Care—Medical Group Development, PHOs, and MSOs

The proliferation of managed care contract activity and the conversion to capitated systems has, in part, led to the development of larger and more comprehensive medical groups, physician hospital organizations (PHOs), management services organizations (MSOs), medical foundations, and fully integrated delivery systems.

THE DESIRE TO PARTICIPATE IN INTEGRATED DELIVERY SYSTEMS

Hospitals

As hospitals began to recognize that their survival depends upon their ability to compete in the managed care arena and to participate in the management of the healthcare service revenues, they became more interested in creating integrated delivery systems which make those goals possible. Hospitals that forego integrated delivery system development face the prospect of having the other participants in the system, physicians, and managed care organizations, treat them merely as cost centers, purchasing hospitals services as they need them. The financial result to hospitals likely would be a downward spiral.

Hospitals are interested in integrated delivery system development because it affords them an opportunity to develop the necessary components to participate in managed care. Over the years, hospitals have faced the legal risks of physician recruitment (including for nonprofit entities), loss of tax-exempt status because of inurement of benefit under the Internal Revenue Service rules, civil and criminal sanctions under Medicare fraud and abuse, and now the inability to bill the Medicare and Medicaid programs where there are certain financial relationships with physicians as a result of the Stark II self-referral prohibitions.

Nonprofit hospitals must be careful of the nature of their physician recruitment activities to ensure that they are consistent with their charitable purposes and that the hospital's funds do not inure to the benefit of the physicians, and thus jeopardize the hospital's tax-exempt status. As a result, hospitals must receive fair value for the money which they are paying to physicians or for any guarantees, and the fair value cannot consist of any payment for the referral of Medicare or Medicaid patients.

A hospital's participation in an integrated delivery system can make the transfer of capital on behalf of physicians possible, strengthen relationships with physicians, and help position the hospital for state and federal healthcare reform. Although the hospital cannot "give" capital to the physicians, with certain forms of integrated delivery systems it can provide the capital to expand or purchase physician practices. Although the physicians may not have an ownership interest in this medical group expansion or development, the physicians indirectly benefit by the creation of a delivery system which can compete in the managed care arena and effectively manage care. If a hospital and physicians work together in an amicable manner in the development and operation of an integrated delivery system and their incentives are aligned, the relationship between them may be strengthened. However, those physicians who are not part of the system, but are or were on the hospital's medical staff, will likely feel alienated, and relationships with them will be adversely affected.

State and federal healthcare reform is an important reason for hospitals to seek to develop integrated delivery systems. Many states are far out in front of the federal government on healthcare reform, and providers in those states have particular incentive to develop integrated delivery systems. Healthcare reform in some form, however, may be enacted by Congress in the future and integrated delivery systems will help position the participants in those systems for healthcare reform.

Physicians

Physicians want to be part of an integrated delivery system because it promises them more managed care contracts and greater access to capital in the development of the system and the expansion of professional practices. Integrated delivery systems also can reduce the cost of physician practices through numerous efficiencies and economies of scale. With more physician practices under management, the costs of managing the practices on a per-unit basis can be reduced. The complexities of management also can be reduced, and better qualified employees can be hired. For example, the quality of an employee who is hired by an integrated delivery system should be high because the system can spread the salary over more physicians and units of service. Furthermore, legal risks associated with physician recruitment activities can be reduced; if physicians are part of a fully integrated system, there should be less legal risk in the areas of Medicare fraud and abuse, antitrust, and inurement. Finally, physicians do not want to be closed out of managed care contracts by not being aligned with a system.

Managed Care Organizations

Managed care organizations also are becoming more interested in integrated delivery system development. Previously, managed care

organizations were merely payors in the system, and now many also
want to be players. Managed care organizations are seeking to align
with or become parts of hospital and physician integrated delivery
systems. In addition, they are seeking to create their own integrated
delivery systems by developing alliances with physicians and accessing hospital care merely through contractual arrangements. Managed care organizations generally have the capital needed for expansion of physician practice activities and, perhaps most importantly,
bring managed care lives to the table. They bring much expertise with
respect to the management of care. However, they do not bring to
the delivery system the high costs associated with hospital care, as
does an asset-based integrated delivery system.

If a managed care organization does not desire to own any part
of the provider delivery system, it may contract with a wide range of
providers as long as it can be assured that those providers will manage
care appropriately in conjunction with the health plan. However,
when a managed care organization seeks to own part of the delivery
system, it may purchase physician practices or employ physicians
from a strong physician group with a history of managed care
experience, and incrementally bring on additional components of
the delivery system as the number of lives in the system warrants.
For example, at one level of lives, additional ambulatory or perinatal
clinics might be developed; at a higher level, an ambulatory surgery
center might be cost-effective. At an even higher level of number of
lives, a short stay hospital might be cost-effective. However, health
plans need to be cautious that they do not jeopardize one of their
greatest assets in the process, flexibility. They should not strive to be
asset-based systems, like hospitals.

MEDICAL GROUP DEVELOPMENT

One of the most important aspects of integrated delivery system
development is the development of a medical group or physician
component of the system which acts like a medical group or a
physician practice division. Physicians are the focus in the manage-

ment of care, and such management of care can be best accomplished with a cohesive group of physicians working together toward that end.

The Independent Practice Association (IPA)

One form of medical group which principally developed during the 1980s was the independent practice association (IPA). In the IPA model, physicians retain their individual practices and their own offices, but they combine into an IPA for the purposes of accessing contracts with payors. Initially, many of the contracts with payors were preferred provider organization (PPO) contracts which paid the physicians on a modified fee-for-service basis either through a discount from the physicians' charges or a fee schedule.

Typically, the hospital assisted the physicians in organizing the IPA to ensure that the hospital had a group of physicians which would participate in the payor contracts which the hospital also would execute with the managed care plans. The hospital often utilized one of its employees to negotiate on behalf of the hospital and the physician group. Inasmuch as there was no sharing of assets and liabilities in such an IPA, it raised significant antitrust issues—the physicians could be accused of price-fixing because they were not part of an integrated group and did not share substantial assets and liabilities. These IPAs served as a means by which the physicians would agree on prices with the health plans.

The problem was exacerbated by the fact that most initial IPAs tended to be inclusive, rather than exclusive. That is, in organizing the IPA, generally a small sign-up fee was required and any physician who wanted to join the IPA who was on the medical staff of a particular hospital might be able to join. As a result, many IPAs consisted of substantial numbers of the medical staff of a hospital, many times well in excess of 50%.

As antitrust scrutiny of these IPAs increased, those that sought to avoid scrutiny by the antitrust regulators sought to employ the messenger concept. In this situation, the IPA used a third party to negotiate its agreements with payors, and each physician would accept or reject the payments offered by the payor. The physicians could suggest that they desired different fees, but the physicians could not conspire with each other to determine the only fees they would extend to or accept from the payor. Most of these messenger arrangements were unwieldy, and many were often ignored by the physicians in the IPA in any event.

As IPAs began to proliferate, many became exclusive rather than inclusive. As they began to accept capitated rates for contracts, it became increasingly important that the physicians who comprised the IPA were able to practice in a cost-effective manner while still maintaining quality of care. Thus, certain physicians might not be asked to join an IPA because their practice patterns were inconsistent with managing care in a cost-effective manner. As a result, newer IPAs became smaller and more exclusive. They also sought to achieve greater degrees of integration for cost containment purposes. Many even sought to capitalize on certain economies of scale by seeking greater degrees of integration.

As managed care and capitation began to proliferate to even a greater extent, and primary care physicians were seen as the focus and gatekeepers for managed care activity, primary care based IPAs began to emerge. These IPAs typically were considerably smaller than the IPAs of the early 1980s, and consisted of primary care physicians often defined to include internists, pediatricians, and obstetricians. These IPAs were able to empower the primary care physicians to take a leadership role, and were more desirable to health plans seeking to contract with physician providers.

Clinic or Group Practice without Walls

Another form of medical group organization is a clinic or group practice without walls. In a clinic without walls model, the physicians combine all or part of their assets and liabilities into a medical group, but they maintain separate offices as if they were in separate practices. Often, the reasons physicians do so is to retain some remnants of private practice or because they are waiting for leases to expire before they combine into a few main sites.

The operation of a clinic without walls is very expensive because of the duplication of many of the resources which are employed by the physicians' offices, including excessive space, reception, billing, and other administrative services. Clinics without walls are often much disfavored by the OIG for Medicare fraud and abuse purposes because of the fear that the physicians might refer to other physicians' patients who are part of the clinic without walls for ancillary services. However, such fears may not be properly founded because the inefficiencies of clinics without walls prohibit them from being true competitors in the long term. To the extent that a clinic without walls has a sufficient degree of integration of practices, the antitrust problems which it might experience are fewer than those experienced by an IPA.

Integrated Medical Group

A fully integrated medical group may be a better vehicle than an IPA or a clinic without walls for the management of care. Integrated medical groups are groups where the physicians have combined their assets and liabilities and generally practice in a few major locations, possibly with some satellite locations. An integrated medical group involves a complete sharing of assets and liabilities in a manner in which the group truly operates as one entity. This form of medical group minimizes antitrust and Medicare fraud and abuse concerns. Inasmuch as the physicians are in close proximity to each other, the ability to manage care is facilitated by their being able to discuss their practices and methods of treatment with other physicians.

However, there is a place for IPAs in the system. It may not be possible to develop an integrated medical group. Certain physicians may be able to practice cost-effective care in an IPA model, and specialty physicians may find the specialty IPA model appealing for a number of reasons (see Chapter 12).

Employment of Physicians

Just as physicians constituting a medical group should have some cohesiveness in the development and operation of the group, a hospital with an integrated delivery system that employs physicians must develop that same cohesiveness to enable the physician employees to practice quality medicine in a cost-effective manner as a division of the integrated delivery system. Thus, employment of physicians by a hospital or other delivery system does not, in itself, necessarily ensure the success of the hospital or other delivery system: the physicians must be able to practice together, as well.

A MEDICAL GROUP AS THE BASIS FOR AN IDS

Once a medical group exists or is formed, it can become the basis for the development of certain forms of integrated delivery systems. For example, a physician organization might join with a hospital to create a third organization called a physician hospital organization (PHO). A management services organization (MSO) might contract with a physician organization which it can manage and/or to which it can deliver services.

PHYSICIAN HOSPITAL ORGANIZATIONS (PHOs)

A physician hospital organization (PHO) is an entity created by a hospital and a physician organization, or physicians and physician groups, to assist in managed care contracting on behalf of the parties. The best PHOs include a physician organization which has its own structure, thus enabling the physicians to tackle issues in the management of care and in the PHO from their perspective. A typical PHO model with a physician organization is set forth in Figure 7-1.

PHOs which have many individual physicians or individual groups participating in the PHO without a central physician organization are often fractionalized, unable to make decisions from the overall physician perspective, and less able to manage care. A PHO model without a separate physician organization is set forth in Figure 7-2.

Although many PHOs have been organized as nonprofit, taxable entities, the better vehicle is a for-profit corporation. The creation of a nonprofit PHO which is funded primarily by a hospital raises substantial issues of Medicare fraud and abuse—and inurement of benefit from the tax-exemption perspective, when physicians are

Figure 7-1
PHO with Physician Organization

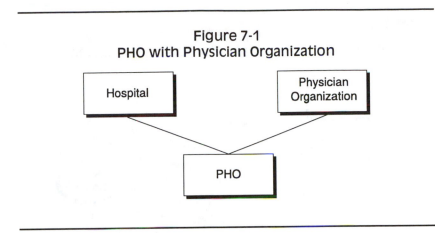

afforded equal control of the assets of the PHO for which they have provided only a small part of the funding, if any, if such control results in a disproportionate benefit to the physicians.

In a for-profit PHO, stock or equity interests in the PHO should be allocated to the hospital and physicians based on the proportion of the assets which they contribute to the PHO. Typically, the hospital contributes cash for its shares, and the physician organization or individual physicians might transfer cash and/or certain parts of the physicians' practice which can be owned by the PHO. These assets might at least include hard assets such as buildings and equipment, and soft assets such as technical know-how, computer software, and other intangibles which are not assets which are directly associated with the operation of the physicians' practice, such as the goodwill associated with the physicians' practice. These other assets generally may only be purchased by the PHO in exchange for stock in the PHO when the PHO can practice medicine in a particular state. PHOs are not often providers of medical services.

The main function of a PHO is to provide managed care contracting services for the hospital and the physicians. A PHO offers a shared governance structure and a recognition that the physicians are an important component of the process of delivering healthcare. PHOs typically also provide utilization review and quality assurance functions. In providing such functions, the PHO needs extensive input

Figure 7-2
PHO without a Separate Physician Organization

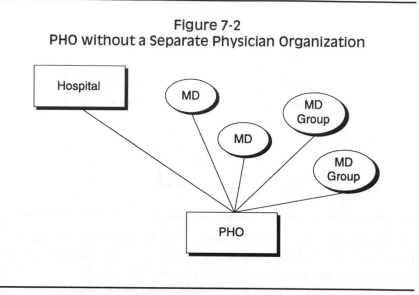

from the physicians in the network to design systems which are workable for the physicians and the hospital. The PHO seeks to align the incentives of the two parties to improve the management of care and its delivery in a more efficient manner. PHOs also employ information systems which can assist in the provision of care. Such systems can track the services rendered to patients in the integrated delivery system and monitor the cost-effectiveness of the care rendered to patients. Such systems should be able to assist in the development of certain practice parameters, protocols, and clinical pathways, and assist in the development of outcomes analysis necessary to ensure the system's efficient operation—and thus appeal to health plans and employer groups.

PHOs have sought to align with other PHOs to offer managed care plans broader physician/hospital networks. Such multiple PHO networks are often known as super PHOs. Such super PHOs must be careful not to be in contravention of the antitrust laws with respect to their operations. Super PHOs which only accept capitation, which do not consist of competing PHOs, and which are nonexclusive likely will be able to survive antitrust scrutiny.

A physician hospital organization is not often considered a sustainable model for integrated delivery system development. The services required by the physician organization are generally greater than those which might typically be provided by a PHO and they do not involve a substantial enough degree of integration to truly align the incentives of the hospital and the physicians. For example, services such as physician practice management, supplies, equipment, space, and employment of nonprofessional and certain professional employees are often important in the continued development and operation of the system. Management services organizations, which should be better capitalized, are generally much better able to render such services to physicians. In addition, those PHOs which are mainly contract vehicles often find it difficult to align incentives because of the interests of the physicians and the hospital compete in this loosely integrated structure.

MANAGEMENT SERVICES ORGANIZATIONS (MSOs)

A management services organization may be defined as an organization which provides services to physicians and physician groups; it also may provide services to a hospital or hospitals. MSOs are sometimes called medical services organizations. An MSO may acquire possession of physicians' tangible assets and certain intangible assets, as with the PHO. An MSO, like a PHO, is generally not a provider or supplier of hospital or medical services for Medicare purposes. Goods and services provided by the MSO should be provided to the physicians and not patients, unless the MSO can practice medicine.

Although only a few states have laws prohibiting the corporate practice of medicine which preclude hospitals and other nonphysician entities from employing physicians, many states have other restrictions on the private practice of medicine. In those states where hospitals are able to employ physicians, many have medical practices acts which seek to exclude nonphysicians from owning shareholder interests in medical groups. As a result, most MSOs which are unable to employ physicians, will have to contract with them. MSOs might provide office space, equipment, furnishings, management information systems, nonprofessional and certain professional personnel, and even provide services to physicians on a turnkey basis. However, when MSOs provide professional personnel for a medical group, the parties need to ensure that they do not run afoul of the Medicare "incident to" rules which only permit physicians to bill for services provided by nonphysician employees where the physician is present at the office location to supervise the nonphysicians, the services are incident to that of the physician's, and the professional personnel are employed by the physician.[3]

MSOs generally are good vehicles for physician recruitment because physicians can contract with the MSO to run their practice. The costs of opening and operating a practice become more certain because MSO services can be offered to the physicians on a flat fee, percentage, or hybrid basis. In addition, the contract with the MSO can be part of a physician recruitment package. However, it should be noted that in the dynamic healthcare market, with its rapid move to managed care, few physicians are likely to be interested in developing private practices which are not part of some larger entity or delivery system positioned to manage care.

An MSO prices its services in a variety of ways, including charging its direct or actual costs of space, equipment, supplies, *etc.*, with a percentage markup or a percentage management fee. The MSO also might charge a percentage of the revenues or collections of the physician organization, but if it is collecting the Medicare or Medicaid services on behalf of the physician organization, it needs to be careful not to run afoul of the Medicare prohibition on an agent charging a percentage of the Medicare or Medicaid payment as a billing or collections fee.[4]

Increasingly, MSOs are charging a portion or percentage of the capitation payments to the medical group as their management fee and sometimes, an incentive fee if the MSO is able to contain costs within certain parameters. Care must be taken to ensure that the fee is a fair one. Often when a system is emerging, it is difficult to determine a fair fee because the number of lives in the system may be very low or nonexistent, and it will not be possible to pay the MSO only a percentage of the capitation fee because many patients will not be capitated. Close attention must be paid to the Medicare fraud and abuse antikickback regulations and, possibly, the Stark II self-referral prohibitions. MSOs affiliated with nonprofit institutions must consider the prohibition against the inurement of benefit in setting MSO fees.

Inasmuch as MSOs can purchase certain assets of physician practices and provide services to physicians, they are a form of joint practice acquisition. Newly recruited, independent physicians can be placed in a central location serviced by the MSO. If the MSO is servicing an IPA, it may have to service physicians in a number of different locations, but it can place the newly recruited physicians in a more efficient practice setting.

MSOs are a step toward the development of more fully integrated delivery systems. They can provide services to a few physicians, a group, or a number of groups of physicians. The range of MSO services and the number of physicians being serviced by the group may increase. The physicians may desire to incorporate into a medical group if they are not currently organized in such a form or, if they are so organized, the group may desire to expand into a multispecialty group. A multispecialty medical group might evolve into a greater form of integration, such as a medical foundation or a fully integrated delivery system.

MSOs can assist in the development of outpatient centers, including ambulatory surgery centers. As healthcare continues to shift to the outpatient setting, such an opportunity becomes more important. Hospitals have not been as efficient as freestanding centers in providing these services because of their high cost structure. Physicians can participate in the delivery of care with the MSO managing their practice, and thus retain a certain degree of autonomy.

MSOs can provide greater access to managed care plans because they offer a mechanism by which the physicians can access managed care contracts. The MSO can jointly negotiate the hospital and physician component of the managed care contract and can act as the agent of the physician in performing utilization review and quality assurance activities.

The MSO can foster practice efficiencies by providing access to better information systems at a lower per physician cost, offering greater technical and management expertise, and assisting the physicians in obtaining better discounts on supplies and inventories. Finally, the MSO leaves some medical practice autonomy with the physicians. The physicians retain their practice and some assets; they merely have a contract with the MSO. The physicians will continue to contract with health plans directly where the MSO cannot hold contracts to provide physician services.

The development and operation of MSOs (and PHOs) raise certain legal issues, particularly those involving Medicare and Medicaid fraud and abuse, tax-exemption, antitrust, corporate practice of medicine or medical practices acts, and perhaps the Stark II self-referral prohibitions. To the extent that an MSO owned all or in part by a hospital does not charge fair market value to the physician for its services, there may be an argument that the MSO is compensating physicians for referrals to the hospital. If the hospital is a nonprofit entity, the amount which is below the fair market value of the MSO services may be seen as a subsidy to the physicians in violation of the IRS prohibition on inurement of benefit.

The Stark II self-referral legislation, known as "The Ethics in Patient Referrals Act," became effective on January 1, 1995. It should be closely reviewed to determine that an MSO's development and operations do not run afoul of this statute. Basically, Stark II prohibits the billing of the Medicare or Medicaid programs for certain designated services, where a physician has an ownership or financial interest in the entity which provides such services, unless one of the exceptions in the statute is met. If the MSO does not provide any designated services, the risk of being in contravention of Stark should be reduced substantially. The inability to bill the Medicare or Medicaid programs likely will be the death knell to any system, and as a result the Stark II law needs to be considered carefully.

Many of the antitrust issues raised by the MSO (or PHO) depend on the nature of the physician organization with which the MSO contracts and the MSO's contracting activities. For example, if the MSO is contracting on behalf of an IPA for fee-for-service payments, the IPA does not have the required degree of integration or risk sharing, and it does not properly employ the messenger concept, the MSO may find it alleged that it is involved in a conspiracy to fix prices because it is coordinating these prices on behalf of the physicians to the managed care plans. In addition, if the MSO serves a considerably high percentage of the physicians in the market, an issue might be raised with respect to the MSO and its contracting physician group attempting to dominate the market in an anticompetitive manner.

An MSO (or PHO) might run afoul of corporate practice of medicine prohibitions or medical practices acts where the entity attempts to purchase the physician practice assets, such as medical records and goodwill associated with a physician practice, or contract directly with a health plan to provide physician services.

The development of MSOs also involves a financial risk. The MSO must be operated as a business, and there should be a business plan for its development and operation. If the MSO is hospital-sponsored, it should not include in the business plan the expectation or value of referrals to the hospital because of the Medicare fraud and abuse implications. The MSO should be able to stand on its own with respect to its operations.

The MSO must generate enough revenue to justify its development and operations. However, as with any new business, part of the MSO's business plan might be that it will lose money for some period of time before it breaks even and later turns a profit. The assumptions on which the business plan are based should be clearly delineated in the plan and should be reasonable.

From the hospital's perspective, even if it owns the MSO, it may have little control over the physician practices depending upon the nature of the contract between the MSO and the hospital. The contracts generally can be terminated at some point in time, and the physicians often have the contract with a health plan. MSOs, however, typically attempt to negotiate long-term contracts with the physician organizations which they serve and they try to limit the availability of early termination clauses. MSOs often invest substantial sums in their development, and most want to ensure that they will recoup those costs.

The following MSO models are often encountered. The model in Figure 7-3, an independent corporation, may be a publicly traded corporation, such as a national physician practice management company (*e.g.*, Caremark Inc.), which provides MSO services to a physician organization through a management services agreement (MSA) for a fee. One of the main services it provides is the negotiation of managed care contracts on behalf of the physician organization and the management of capitated revenues. The fee the MSO charges may be based on the management company's cost of providing services, plus a markup, a budgeted amount, or a percentage of revenues. It also may be based on the capital expended by the MSO plus a return on capital, and it even might include an incentive payment if the MSO is able to keep the costs per member per month to a certain level. The MSO often seeks to take an assignment of the

Figure 7-3
Independent MSO

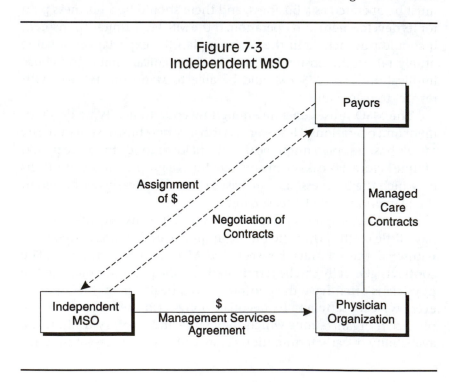

managed care revenues, retain a portion for its fee, and perhaps make payments to other entities on behalf of the physician organization. In states where fee splitting is not permitted, and/or nonphysician professional corporations cannot practice medicine, the MSA should not be used as a means to split fees or medical group profits.

MSOs may seek to manage large medical groups which have worked together and under capitation, as well as smaller, developing medical groups; or they may even seek to develop medical groups in conjunction with their MSO operations. Usually they seek to enter into long-term contracts with physician groups to enable them to recoup their investment. Often they even seek transactions with captive medical groups; that is, where the owner of the medical group which the MSO is managing is or becomes an employee of the MSO. Of course, such an arrangement is not necessary in states where the owners of the MSO can own all or part of the medical group.

Most national MSOs are in business to make a profit. Their ability to be successful depends on their ability to keep the costs of the physicians' practice as low as possible, enable the practice to maximize revenue, and to make a profit from their operation of the practice.

In the model shown in Figure 7-4, a hospital owns all the stock of the MSO and operates it as a subsidiary. In many hospital-owned MSOs, the MSO seeks to charge the physician as little as possible for MSO services. However, such an MSO must ensure that it charges the physicians fair value for its services to ensure that it is not in violation of the Medicare fraud and abuse laws, possibly the Stark II self-referral laws; or, if the hospital owner of the MSO is a nonprofit, tax-exempt entity, that it does not violate the IRS prohibition on inurement of benefit.

In the model shown in Figure 7-5, physicians own the stock of the MSO. They may consist of all or part of the physicians who are receiving services from the MSO. In a physician-owned MSO where the physicians who own the MSO are not identical to the physicians receiving services from the MSO, an inherent conflict exists. The physicians who own the MSO want to make a profit from the operations. Of course, however, the more the physician-owned MSO

Figure 7-4
Hospital-Owned MSO

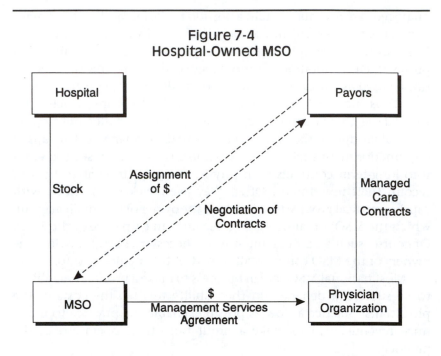

charges the physicians for their MSO service, the less money the physicians receiving those services realize.

Inasmuch as the model shown in Figure 7-6 contemplates joint hospital and physician ownership in the MSO, its organizational structure is similar to the PHO. Although this MSO model may be preferred by some because it assures shared governance by the hospital and physician owners, it often is difficult for physicians to invest the necessary capital to purchase their equity interest in the MSO. The physicians, however, might sell their hard assets and soft assets capable of being owned by an MSO, such as technical know-how, to the MSO in exchange for their equity interest. MSOs, however, generally have large capital requirements because they invest in management information systems and assets necessary to assist in the operation and management of physician practices.

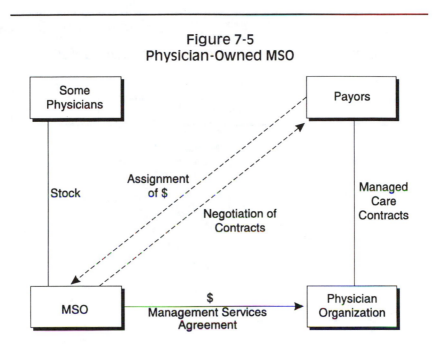

Figure 7-5
Physician-Owned MSO

A managed care organization (MCO) MSO may be organized as a subsidiary of a MCO or as a division of a for-profit MCO. Figure 7-7 sets forth the subsidiary model. Managed care organizations are seeking to develop MSOs to ensure that they have adequate provider networks to service their beneficiaries and that they are players in integrated delivery system development. Managed care organizations have the necessary capital to develop and operate MSOs. They may offer as well tested information systems and the experience of managing care. In addition, such MSOs are particularly attractive to physicians because they can bring managed care lives to the system. However, the MCO MSO model has an inherent conflict—payors may be disinclined to contract with an MCO MSO because the MCO is a competitor to the payors.

Figure 7-6
Joint Venture Hospital and Physician-Owned MSO

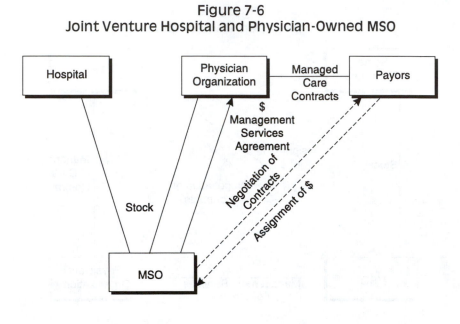

CONCLUSION

The proliferation of capitated managed care contracting activity has led to the development of more medical group formation, the emergence and development of PHOs and MSOs to assist in managed care contracting, and the alignment of physician and hospital incentives. As there are myriad models, the particular situation and relationship among the parties should dictate the structures they employ.

Figure 7-7
Managed Care Organization Owned MSO

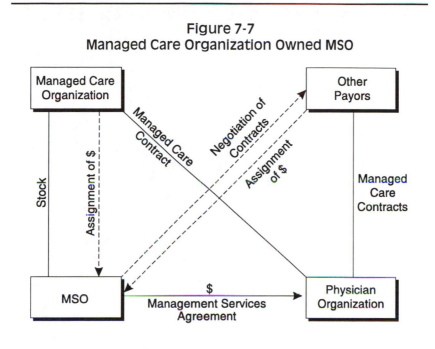

8

More Fully Integrated Structures to Manage Care— Medical Foundations and Fully Integrated Delivery Systems, Including the Physician Equity Model

Medical groups, PHOs, and MSOs are not fully integrated delivery systems in and of themselves, absent certain other relationships. For example, a medical group which owns a hospital can be a fully integrated delivery system, but absent such hospital ownership, it would not be a fully integrated delivery system. In fact, a medical group which owns a hospital is known as the physician equity model of integration, a well-known form of integrated delivery system, discussed later in this chapter.

In those states in which PHOs or MSOs can own physician practices or practice medicine, it might be possible for them to own the hospital and the physician practice assets and provide hospital and physician services. However, in such an event the PHO or MSO has really evolved into a more fully integrated form of delivery system and is no longer operating merely as a PHO or MSO.

MEDICAL FOUNDATIONS

A more fully integrated IDS is a medical foundation, affiliated with a hospital, which is a nonprofit corporation exempt from taxation under Section 501(c)(3) of the Internal Revenue Code which employs or contracts with physicians and/or physician groups to provide medical services. The activities of a medical foundation might include the operation of outpatient clinics and facilities which it owns or leases, the furnishing of equipment and supplies for the provision of medical services, and the conducting of medical research and health education. Typically, medical foundations employ nonphysician individuals to operate their facilities and either employ or contract with physician individuals to provide medical services at the foundation. Physician executives, however, are taking a greater role in the operation and management of medical foundations and more fully integrated delivery systems.

The medical foundation contracts with the managed care plan directly, and it can perform all those activities which might typically be performed by physician practices, including billing, collections, procurement of insurance, and administrative and general services. The medical foundation is essentially a physician practice operated and managed by a nonprofit entity.

Medical foundations can be very good vehicles for physician recruitment. They can hire or independently contract with physicians for a set fee. There is no need for physicians to develop separate practices. However, the physicians should be operating in an efficient division of the medical foundation for the foundation to be cost-effective.

The medical foundation is a true form of physician practice acquisition because the medical foundation actually purchases the physician practice. It is an advanced step toward an integrated delivery system. Once the medical foundation is established, it only needs to align or affiliate with a hospital to develop an integrated delivery system which includes both a hospital and physician component.

A medical foundation provides a greater degree of security for physicians with little or no capital risk. If it is affiliated with a hospital, managed care contracting and the development of outpatient centers are substantially easier. It can achieve greater economies of scale, and operates as a charitable organization.

To obtain its tax-exempt status, the IRS generally requires that a medical foundation be organized for charitable purposes; none of its assets can inure to the benefit of private individuals and it cannot provide more than incidental benefits to private individuals. If the foundation has a hospital component, it must maintain an open emergency department and an open medical staff. In addition, it generally must conduct medical education and research. The Board of Directors of the medical foundation should be community-based and no more than 20% of its membership may be physician insiders. In addition, physician insiders cannot be involved in determining their own compensation from the medical foundation. However, the 20% limitation does not extend to all physicians—only those who are insiders with some direct or indirect financial relationship with the foundation.

When a medical foundation acquires physician practice assets, it must acquire those assets for no more than fair market value, and the purchase price must be based on independent appraisals and arm's length negotiations between the parties. No part of the acquisition price should be for any possible referrals to the hospital component of the integrated delivery system.

The IRS requires that fair market value be based on the business enterprise value (BEV) to a likely purchaser, which is determined after subtracting the amount of long-term debt from the capital structure, leaving shareholder or partner equity, known as the enterprise's net worth. The IRS requires that three methods of estimating the BEV be included in all appraisals with applications for tax-exempt status for integrated delivery systems. They are the income approach, the market approach, and the cost approach.

In addition, the IRS requires that the income approach valuation should use an aftertax, not a pretax, cash-flow assumption, or an inflated value could be created in the seller. Further, the revenues in the valuation should not consider revenues generated from self-referrals which would be prohibited by the Stark II self-referral law.

Any committees created to consider the business or charitable aspects of the foundation's operations should be independent and representative of the community. Committees which solely consider the clinical or professional aspects of healthcare can have an unlimited number of physicians.

A medical foundation might be organized in a number of ways, described next. In the model shown in Figure 8-1, the hospital owner controls the foundation and it seeks to align the incentives of the physicians in the subsidiary organization with the hospital. (This model is similar to the hospital-controlled integrated delivery system model shown in Figure 8-9.)

In the model shown in Figure 8-2, one corporate entity operates both the hospital and the physician practice divisions. Such a model results in a greater integration than the prior foundation model (Figure 8-1). It is easier to align the incentives of the hospital and the physicians, and legal issues are minimized because both the hospital and the physicians are part of one entity.

The model shown in Figure 8-3 is merely a means by which a nonprofit foundation can operate a physician practice division.

Figure 8-1
Hospital-Owned or Controlled Foundation

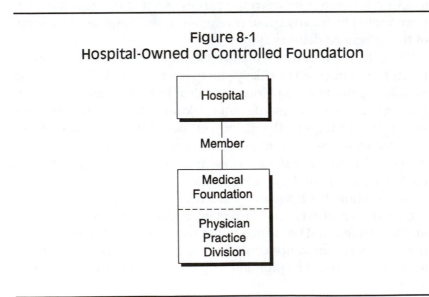

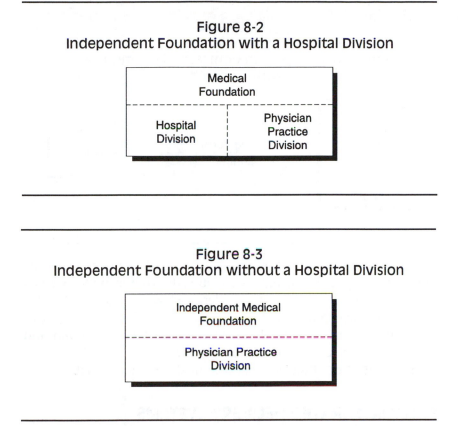

Figure 8-2
Independent Foundation with a Hospital Division

Figure 8-3
Independent Foundation without a Hospital Division

Without a hospital component, it is not a fully integrated delivery system. However, it may contract with a hospital to replicate an integrated delivery system. If it does so, it will want to ensure that the incentives of the physicians are aligned with a hospital with which it contracts to develop a true form of integrated delivery systems, or it will want to treat the hospital as a cost center. Figure 8-4 sets forth the situation of an independent medical foundation without a hospital division with a long-term contractual relationship with a hospital.

In Figure 8-4, the independent foundation contracting with the hospital on a long-term contractual arrangement may seek to replicate the physician equity model for the physicians by treating the

Figure 8-4
Independent Foundation without a Hospital Division, but with a Long-Term Contractual Relationship with a Hospital

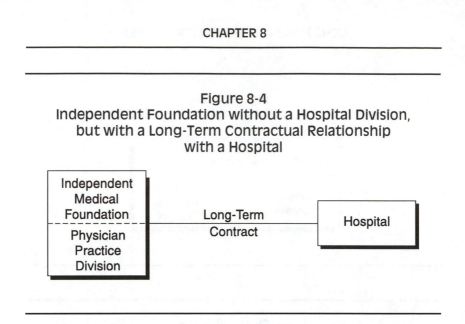

hospital as a cost center. This model, however, does not achieve true integration because the medical foundation does not own the hospital.

Medical foundations face considerable legal issues, but they are somewhat easier to resolve than those in the PHO or MSO context. The major legal issues involve Medicare and Medicaid fraud and abuse, Stark self-referral prohibitions, tax-exemption, antitrust, and corporate practice of medicine and/or medical practices acts.

FULLY INTEGRATED DELIVERY SYSTEMS

An integrated delivery system is an organization, or group of affiliated organizations, which provides physician and hospital services to patients. More integrated or sophisticated systems might provide additional services, such as home health, hospice, skilled nursing, preventative medicine, mental health, rehabilitation, and long-term care. It does not necessarily include a payment component such as a managed care organization, but it may. If it is nonprofit, and it wants to be exempt from taxation under IRS Section 501(c)(3), it will need to at least meet the same tests as the medical foundation discussed above. The IRS takes the position that each entity within the integrated delivery system will have its tax status determined separately based on its own individual characteristics and activities.

Integrated delivery systems are known by a number of names, including integrated healthcare system, integrated healthcare delivery system, integrated healthcare organizations, and physician-hospital organization (PHO). The latter nomenclature is confusing, however, in light of the earlier discussion of PHOs, which are mainly managed care contracting vehicles.

Integrated delivery systems make possible the development of a unified, strategic plan. Services are provided in the best possible setting for patient care and for reimbursement systems. There is less duplication of services, and therefore costs should be less.

The allocation of capital can be based on the maximum benefit to the community. Physician and hospital priorities should be considered together and prioritized accordingly. However, in light of past relationships between hospitals and physicians, it is particularly necessary to achieve a delicate balance of these priorities. In the past, many hospitals and their medical staffs have mistrusted each other. These barriers must be overcome to effectively develop and operate an integrated delivery system.

Integrated delivery systems facilitate physician recruitment and retention. Physicians can be paid their fair value for providing services. However, a system's ability to do so well will depend upon the profitability of the system. Obviously a system which eventually loses money may have difficulty paying physician salaries and/or guarantees.

Fully integrated delivery systems offer an attractive option for managed care plans. By contracting with the IDS, both hospital and physician services are obtained. An IDS is a form of one-stop shopping. Theoretically, the health plan does not need to concern itself with the allocation of the capitated dollar. If it capitates the provider network, it should be assumed that its beneficiaries will receive the necessary hospital and physician services for a set fee. However, the managed care plan should ensure that the system with which it is contracting is viable and solvent and that it can manage care.

Integrated delivery systems can maximize physicians' incentives to deliver the best quality medicine to patients in the most effective manner, and are an excellent model for competing. IDS can develop quality tracking systems and work with the physicians in the system to successfully implement them. In addition, they can assist in the development of practice parameters, protocols, and clinical pathways designed to facilitate the delivery of care in a cost-effective manner. Integrated system development often strains physician relationships, in part because the physician compensation issues are complicated.

Descriptions of some possible models of integrated delivery systems follow. In IDS models one and two (Figures 8-5 and 8-6), the physicians typically are employees of the entity, but they operate as a division. The employment by an entity or a hospital of a few primary care physicians or specialists, however, will not result in the development of a truly integrated delivery system. The physician employees must be organized in such a manner, with sufficient critical mass, that they can be the physician practice division of the integrated delivery system managing care.

Model one, Figure 8-5, includes a managed care component which affords the integrated delivery system the ability to directly contract with employer groups. It may be difficult for an IDS to include a managed care component as a division of its corporate entity because of state regulatory requirements which might necessitate the MCO being organized as a separate corporation; for non-profit IDS, the MCO may need to be organized as a separate corporation because it may not be able to obtain an IRC § 501(c)(3) status, but only an IRC § 501(c)(4) status.

In IDS models three and four (Figures 8-7 and 8-8), the parent holding company either owns the hospital and the physician practice corporation (and the managed care company, if it is part of the IDS) by virtue of stock ownership or controls it by nonprofit membership. In some states, such ownership of the physician practice corporation may not be possible because the shares of the physician practice organization might be held only by physicians, or because physicians may not be able to practice in a nonprofit corporate form. However, in states where such ownership structures are not prohibited, the parent holding company model can be an effective form of integrated delivery system provided the boards of the parent holding

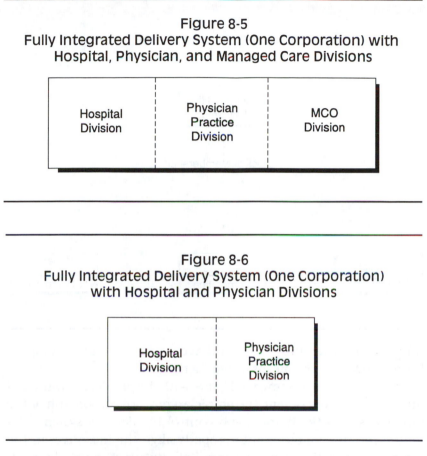

Figure 8-5
Fully Integrated Delivery System (One Corporation) with Hospital, Physician, and Managed Care Divisions

| Hospital Division | Physician Practice Division | MCO Division |

Figure 8-6
Fully Integrated Delivery System (One Corporation) with Hospital and Physician Divisions

| Hospital Division | Physician Practice Division |

company, the hospital, the physician practice corporation, and the managed care company (if it is part of the IDS) are appropriately constituted, the physicians have substantial input, and the entities work together in true integration.

In the IDS model shown in Figure 8-9, the hospital-controlled integrated delivery system model, the hospital owns the physician practice corporation. This model only would be possible in states where nonphysicians can own or be a nonprofit corporate member of a physician practice corporation. This model is fully integrated, as the hospital seeks to align the incentives of the physicians with the

Figure 8-7
Parent Holding Company Model IDS with
Managed Care Component

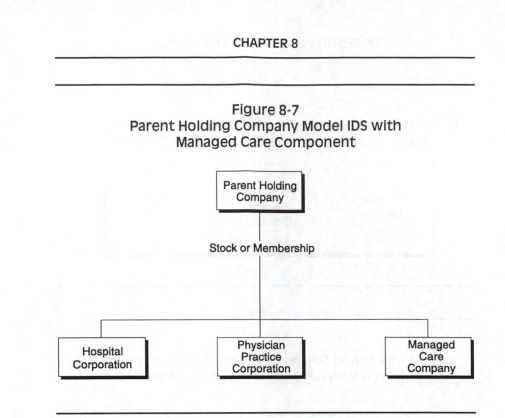

hospital. However, the physicians have no real control because the hospital owns all the means of production.

In the IDS model shown in Figure 8-10, the physician-controlled integrated delivery system, the physician practice corporation or the physicians own the hospital and control the delivery system. The physicians are in a position to properly align the incentives in the system because they own the hospital, and treat it merely as an operating entity complementary to the physician practices. This model is typically known as "the physician equity model." Although much touted in the industry as an ideal model, the ability of physicians to develop such a model is limited because their access to capital generally is limited. However, many physicians soon realize that it is not the ownership of a hospital itself which results in the creation of a physician equity model, but the ability of the physicians to have a health plan pay the physicians for hospital services whether or not they own a hospital. In a capitated environment, subject to state insurance laws as noted above, a physician group may be able to take

Figure 8-8
Parent Holding Company Model IDS without
Managed Care Component

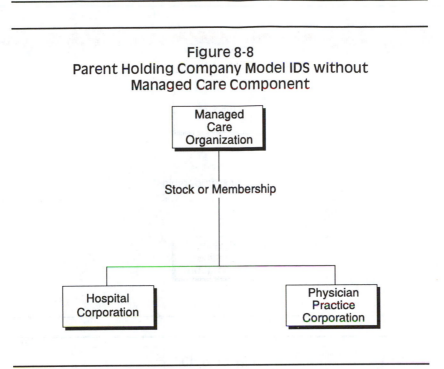

hospital capitation payments and subcapitate or pay a hospital for such services on a modified fee-for-service basis. In a fee-for-service model, most payors generally pay only the licensed hospital facility for services rendered to the patient, not some intermediate entity which does not own a hospital.

In the IDS Model shown in Figure 8-11, a managed care organization controls the integrated delivery system. The managed care organization may own the hospital provider and the physician practice organization, employ the physicians directly in some form of staff model, or contract on a long-term basis with the hospital and physicians. If the managed care organization-controlled integrated delivery system is a closed system, its physician and hospital providers only render services to enrollees of the managed care organization. If the managed care organization controlled integrated delivery system is an open system, its physician and hospital providers may render services to patients who are not enrollees of the managed care

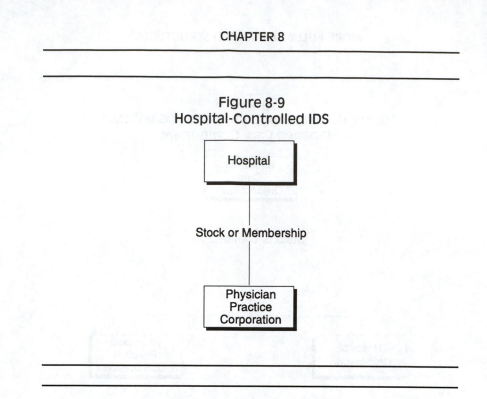

Figure 8-9
Hospital-Controlled IDS

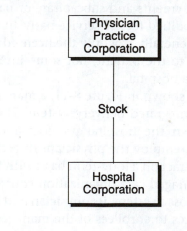

Figure 8-10
Physician-Controlled IDS (the "Physician Equity" Model)

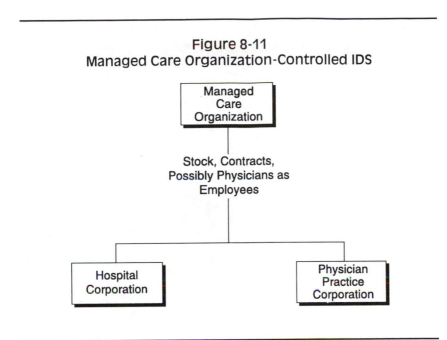

Figure 8-11
Managed Care Organization-Controlled IDS

organization. Of course, managed care organizations might be reluctant to contract with managed care organization-controlled integrated delivery systems for competitive reasons, but managed care companies and providers often have numerous alliances, many of which potentially conflict.

CONCLUSION

No one form of foundation or fully integrated delivery system model works in each instance. The goals and objectives of the parties are of paramount importance in designing an IDS. The models are merely a starting point. The parties will want to design a system which best aligns the incentives of the parties and positions them to manage and deliver quality care in a cost-effective manner.

9

Physician Compensation

The alignment of incentives is important in the success of managed care and integrated delivery systems. An important component in such an alignment is the method by which physicians are compensated. As noted above, capitation is generally thought to be the preferred method of payment to physicians to ensure the delivery of cost-effective healthcare services. The managed care plan typically pays the physician organization, the hospital, or the integrated delivery system the capitated amount. From that fixed amount of money, the individual physician is compensated. This chapter discusses a variety of methods by which the physician organization, hospital, or integrated delivery system receiving the physician capitation payments might compensate the individual physician.

FEE-FOR-SERVICE BASIS

Physicians may be compensated on a fee-for-service basis. As used in this chapter, compensation on a fee-for-service basis means a payment to the physician each time the physician has an encounter with the patient. The payment may be a percentage discount from the physician's charges or an amount set forth in a fee schedule. Although initially with the development of capitation, it was thought advisable to pay the individual primary care physicians for their services on a capitated basis, increasingly paying such physicians on a fee-for-service basis is becoming a desired method of compensation. Of course, their overall fee-for-service payments are limited by the capitation payments allocable to the primary care physicians in the aggregate.

Many capitated systems pay the specialty physicians on a fee-for-service basis. As discussed above, these physicians order the most expensive tests and perform the expensive procedures. As a result, the capitation of such individual providers can be an important consideration in containing the costs of a system. However, there likely will be a number of physicians for whom there may not be enough lives to capitate the specialist to reduce his or her risk. As a result, fee-for-service payments may remain a payment mechanism for some individual specialists.

WITHHOLDS/RISK POOLS

Although withholds and risk pools are not actually a compensation system, they are used in conjunction with other compensation methods to create new compensation systems. For example, where the primary care physicians are ultimately subject to an overall cap on their compensation because they are in a capitated system, but the individual physician compensation method is fee-for-service, a withhold can help ensure that the system will be able to pay the individual physicians on a fee-for-service basis by retaining the monies withheld in a risk pool for later distribution.

Once the fee-for-service payment schedule is adopted, a certain percentage of each payment can be withheld from the individual physicians to ensure that there will be sufficient monies available during a particular period (such as a quarter, half, or whole year) to continue to make the fee-for-service payments. If, at the end of the period, monies remain in the withhold fund or risk pool which have not been used for fee-for-service payments, and all claims to the fund for the year have been accounted for, these remaining monies may be paid to the physicians.

Withholds are often used in conjunction with payments to specialists on a fee-for-service basis. Such withholds may be particularly important as a means to ensure that there are sufficient monies available to pay the specialists because their utilization of services through the ordering of costly tests and performance of procedures likely will vary to a greater extent than that of the primary care physicians.

Withholds also can be used in conjunction with many compensation methods, including capitation, payment pursuant to a formula, point system, discretionary method, or salary. A percentage of the capitation payment might be withheld from individual physicians if all the physicians in the network for whose services they are financially responsible are not paid on a capitated basis. In such an instance, the physicians responsible for all the physician payments will want to ensure that there are sufficient monies available to pay all the IBNRs.

Risk pools are often used as an incentive mechanism to ensure proper utilization. If monies remain in the risk pool after a certain period of time, they are returned to the physicians, and possibly a portion also to the health plan and the hospital, pursuant to some formula.

CAPITATION

An individual physician or a group of physicians providing services in the network can be compensated by capitation. The capitated physicians receive a fixed payment pmpm to provide physician services. Primary care physicians may be capitated for all physician services, with the result that they will contract with specialty physicians for specialty services; or the primary care physicians might only be capitated through the network for the primary care services they can provide.

Specialty physicians might be subcapitated by the primary care physicians or the network or capitated directly by the health plan. Through the development of specialty medical groups contracting with numerous health plans and networks, an increasing number of specialists should be able to increase the number of lives for which they are responsible, with the result that they will limit their overall risk of providing services for a capitated payment.

FORMULAS

There are numerous formulas by which physicians can be paid in a managed care network. These formulas include those based on overhead allocations, productivity, minimization of costs, or some combination thereof.

Overhead Allocation Formulas

With an overhead allocation formula, the overhead in the group or network associated with that physician's individual practice is chargeable against the revenues associated with that physician's individual practice. Overhead might be allocated based on percentage of revenues, number of encounters, hours of practice, or any other method which the parties desire. The revenues associated with the physician might be the payments on a fee-for-service, capitated, or other basis, plus any payments from withholds or risk pools.

Productivity Formulas

Many productivity formulas are based on the assumption that all the services which the physician performed were necessary. That is, a physician in the network would have to have had a patient encounter, and be paid more because he or she works harder by seeing more patients than another physician. Such a system might include compensation to a physician which is based all or in part on the fact that the physician may have experienced X encounters, and there are Y primary care encounters; as a result, the physician should receive X/Y of the primary care payments. Such productivity based formulas work best in a capitated system, where there are restrictions to ensure proper utilization. It is particularly important in a productivity based system to ensure that the physicians are in no way compensated for overutilization. In fact, in productivity based payment systems, physicians might be penalized for both over- and underutilization.

Minimization of Cost Formulas

A compensation formula based on the physician's minimization of cost is difficult to devise and administer because the compensation should be based on the minimization of those costs which the physician can control, and payment should not be made for minimizing the treatment of patients or enrollees. A determination should first be made of those costs which the physician can control, and the formula at least based in part on same. Care should be taken to ensure that utilization is appropriate.

Hybrid Formulas

Overhead, productivity, and cost considerations can all be part of formula compensation in conjunction with each other, or any of the two can be combined. In addition, other factors could be included in the formula. For example, in a faculty practice compensation plan, the physicians also would receive compensation for their teaching and research activities.

POINT SYSTEM

Many physician compensation systems are based on points allocated to physicians. Points might be accumulated for years of practice, years with the group, special experience, participation in call schedules, coverage, hours worked, staffing clinics in less desirable areas, teaching, research, or other functions. The physician's compensation may be based on his or her percentage of the total number of points in the system times the compensation payments for the period, *e.g.,* a month. A certain number of points may be reserved for bonuses at the end of the year.

DISCRETIONARY

Physician compensation systems may be discretionary. That is, physician compensation may be set by a board or committee based on a number of factors, including a budget of the anticipated revenues and expenses for the year, the expected productivity of the physician, and the physician's value to the group. Such systems result in great uncertainty and anxiety for the physicians, but are dynamic in that they can readily adapt to changes in revenues and the expenses associated with the physician's practice. Discretionary payment methods are often used for the payment of bonuses to physicians.

SALARY

An often employed method of physician compensation is the salary. Physicians' employees are typically paid on this basis. The salary may be set within a range of fair market value salaries for the physician. Payment of the physicians on a fair market value basis is particularly important if a nonprofit entity is paying the physicians. In addition, a medical group will not want to pay excessive salaries in any event because of its fiscal constraints. With a salary, a physician employee typically will have a job description, expected performance targets, and possibly a written employment contract.

Many people believe that physicians do not make good employees, particularly those who are now joining networks or becoming employees of hospitals, if they were accustomed to fee-for-service medicine and operating their own offices. The physicians who wanted to be employees of health plans, hospitals, and large medical groups are already employees of such entities. The physicians who did not want to be such employees, but who wanted to own and manage their own practices, are now often being thrust into practice settings where they are employees—practice settings they neither chose nor desired. The motivation of such physicians is pivotal in the successful management of care and system development. An important consideration is how to provide that motivation.

PRODUCTIVITY OR INCENTIVE BONUSES

Motivation of physicians might be accomplished with a productivity or incentive bonus. The formula for such could be based on a similar analysis as a productivity compensation payment mechanism formula. The incentives may be based on the productivity of the physician component of an integrated delivery system or the system as a whole. It also may be based on keeping costs of treatment of patients down to a specific cost pmpm. However, one must be careful in designing such productivity bonuses to ensure that they do not run afoul of any prohibitions on payments to physicians for underutilization.

The more effective salary, plus incentive bonus systems, might peg the physicians' salaries at some amount below market value, *e.g.* 85%, and the percentage bonus should be substantial, perhaps increasing the physicians' compensation by as much as 30 to 40%. The incentive should be meaningful enough to ensure a positive effect on the physicians.

The incentive bonus can be based on the overall performance of the physician division, the individual physician's performance, or a combination of the two. Better compensation systems likely will include both elements of an incentive systems.

AMBULATORY PAYMENT GROUPS

As noted in Chapter 3, an emerging payment alternative is payment based on ambulatory payment groups. Payment by APGs to specialists may become a desired method of compensation for those systems which have an insufficient number of lives to capitate the specialists. The APG payment methodology can help control the utilization of services, but does not require a minimum number of lives to be successfully implemented. If their use is successful, they may even rival capitation as the compensation method of choice. It, however, is too early to determine whether such will be the case.

CONCLUSION

No one physician compensation system is necessarily better than the others. Compensation systems should be designed to meet the needs of the particular physicians who are being compensated and in a manner which best aligns the incentives of the parties. In addition, any compensation system should be dynamic—that is, it should be flexible and revised as often as necessary (even yearly) to accommodate the needs of the physicians and the network.

10

Managing Care

Although it is generally recognized that the management of care to minimize the cost per member per month is the objective in a managed care system and for integrated delivery systems, how this objective is achieved is less understood. It is not simply the assignment of a primary care physician to an enrollee where the primary care physician seeks to ensure that the enrollee's services are limited, and that access to a specialist is restricted. The management of care may involve the implementation of practice parameters, protocols, clinical or critical pathways, and outcomes analysis. In developing such tools to manage care, and in the overall management of care, the employment of management information systems is important. The parties must have a commitment to managing care, and there must be a sufficient capitated population to ensure that the parties are able to manage care.

PRACTICE PARAMETERS

Practice parameters are practice guidelines which have been systematically developed to assist the physician and patient in making decisions about the appropriate course of treatment for specific clinical indications. The parameters of physicians' practices need to be better standardized through the development of and adherence to practice parameters that focus on cost-effective, quality care. Prior to implementing such parameters or guidelines, it is helpful to know how they were developed, by whom, and whether they are supported by empirical data. For physicians developing their own practice parameters, any scientific evidence or study which supports their position will help to minimize the legal risk for the employment of such parameters.

It is just as important to ensure that excessive tests and procedures are not performed as it is to ensure that needed tests and procedures are not limited. The latter could be even more detrimental to a patient's well-being and to keeping the overall cost of the system down. The idea should be to strive toward a healthier population, with the result that the cost of treating that population diminishes. Obviously, if the population for which the physician is responsible is healthier because of the practice patterns of the physician, the physicians and the integrated delivery system will realize more net revenues because the costs will be less.

PROTOCOLS

It also is important to develop specific treatment protocols or plans which maximize the efficiency of treatment of a particular patient. Such protocols should be developed and implemented with substantial physician input and support, to ensure that they are not only the standard of care, but also that they become effective tools in the management of care and in its cost-effective delivery.

CLINICAL OR CRITICAL PATHWAYS

The development of clinical or critical pathways also is important in the management of care. These pathways generally are strictly defined and procedure-specific. They describe key events in the process of patient care which physicians believe will result in optimal quality at a minimal cost. They should be available to the physicians at the appropriate clinical time. It is important to determine the best and most efficient course of treatment and means by which the physician can provide the best quality of care in the most cost-effective manner.

By developing clinical pathways, it is possible to develop more cost-effective modes of treatment.

Standards also may be developed which identify a range of acceptable care and which may be consulted in the confirmation of diagnoses. Such standards are often known as boundary guidelines because they propose to set boundaries in the range of care.

OUTCOMES ANALYSIS

It also is important to track outcomes over time to ensure that the treatment modalities employed are leading to the best outcomes, and to support the basis for the assertion that a provider or provider group has rendered quality care. Employer groups will become increasingly interested in outcomes analysis data from providers. Such information should make the comparability of provider systems on a quality basis easier to determine. Provider systems which achieve favorable outcomes will be more attractive to health plans and employer groups because their beneficiaries or employees will be healthier and should experience less lost time from work. In addition, such provider systems should be less costly and will be able to offer lower rates to health plans and employer groups.

MANAGEMENT INFORMATION SYSTEMS

A management information system is important in developing, implementing, and monitoring practice parameters, protocols, clinical pathways, and tracking outcomes. It should be continually updated and designed to ensure that the system provides usable information for the providers, and assists them in developing the tools to practice more cost-effective, quality medicine.

The ideal information system would be user- or physician-friendly. A physician might handwrite on an electronic pad, speak into a voice-activated system, or key in the symptoms, diagnosis, and proposed plan of treatment for a particular patient. The system might advise the physician if any tests have been ordered which perhaps should not have been for a patient with certain symptoms, or whether he or she has failed to order any tests which should have been ordered. The system might advise the physician what additional symptoms or indications need to be present to justify the ordering of the additional test. If they are present, the physician indicates that they are, and proceeds to order them. If not, the physician will have to justify ordering such tests.

If the patient is admitted to the hospital, the physician should be able to access the patient's electronic medical record in his or her office. By accessing the medical record, the physician can ascertain important information about a patient's progress, whether it is necessary for the physician to visit the patient that day and when, and whether the physician should order additional tests or procedures. The patient's length of stay in the hospital might be monitored in conjunction with certain benchmarks for patients who have been admitted with the same diagnosis.

From the information obtained from the physician's encounter with the patient and the hospital, it may be possible over time to revise practice parameters, protocols, and clinical pathways to be more effective. In addition, such data can help develop the outcomes analysis necessary to demonstrate to health plans and employer groups the true effectiveness of the system.

COMMITMENT TO MANAGING CARE

It should be noted that even the development of the best practice parameters, protocols, and clinical pathways will not lead to the cost-effective management of care unless the physicians who are responsible for adopting and implementing them agree with them and are committed to managing care. The management of care involves a mind set or a method of practice different from that for fee-for-service medicine. A physician in a fee-for-service environment measures success based on the number of encounters and/or procedures with patients. A physician in a capitated managed care environment measures success based on the wellness of the patient population for which he or she is responsible, the maximization of capitated revenues, and the minimization of costs.

A SUFFICIENT CAPITATED POPULATION

It is not easy for physicians to manage care when they only have a few patients under capitation or they have a mix of few capitated and many fee-for-service patients. At some point, however (*e.g.*, 30 to 40% managed care patients), physicians are able to practice as if they are in a managed care environment.

It also is important for physicians to stop thinking in terms of what their charges would have been for a particular patient had that patient been a fee-for-service patient. First of all, that patient is not a fee-for-service patient, but a managed care patient. Second, even if the patient was a fee-for-service patient, it is unlikely that the physician is being paid full fees in any event; rather the physician is more likely being paid pursuant to a fee schedule or discount from charges, which results in a significant discount from "usual and customary fees." Third, physicians should be thinking in terms of fair compensation for the lives for which the they are responsible and the patients they treat. If a physician is responsible for 1,500 lives and receives a capitation payment of $15 per month, that physician's gross revenues per year will be $270,000. After paying expenses, what is the physician's take-home pay, and is that consistent with what the physician might have made in a fee-for-service world? If it is, the physician probably has done very well because, under fee-for-service agreements, the physician's income is likely to decline.

What about the hospital's ability to manage care? It needs to stop thinking in terms of the census each day. In a capitated environment, hospital administration does not want the hospital to be full; it wants to have sufficient patients to be operational and maintain the necessary JCAHO accreditation, but the hospital should want a healthy population which requires fewer hospital services because the use of those services costs the hospital money if it is being paid a fixed amount pmpm for hospital care. This is a significant step for the hospital, however, because many hospitals view success as having their beds full and delivering as many services as possible. Success in a managed care environment is just the opposite: being as empty as possible, but maintaining accreditation and delivering as few services as possible.

As discussed above, managing care also means managing inappropriate underutilization of hospital facilities and physician services. Care must be managed with wellness in mind.

A WORKABLE MODEL

To be able to appropriately manage care, it is necessary for the parties to have a model which is workable for them and which best facilitates the management of care. Although many models seek to manage care by having the primary care physician assume as much of a patient's care as possible, there is some thought that perhaps the specialist should take a greater role. Patients with a specific injury or disease might be managed better by a specialist, in coordination with the primary care physician. As noted above, the emerging ambulatory payment group compensation systems also may be employed to ensure a workable model. Newer models will continue to emerge as physicians explore ways to best manage a patient's care in a managed care environment.

CONCLUSION

Managing care involves more than merely capitating physicians and hospitals. Practice parameters, protocols, clinical or critical pathways, and outcomes analysis also are important in managing care. Care cannot be appropriately managed in a cost-effective manner unless management information systems are employed to assist in doing so. In addition, the parties must have a demonstrated commitment to managing care, and if a capitated system is implemented, there should be a sufficient capitated population.

11

Credentialing

Credentialing is the means by which it is determined whether a physician will be able to obtain privileges to practice at a hospital, to render services to the patients of a health plan, or to practice with a medical group or in a network. The granting of privileges by a hospital and hospital credentialing is beyond the scope of this book. This chapter addresses credentialing by managed care plans, medical groups, and networks.

THE PROCESS OF CREDENTIALING

The process of credentialing by the managed care plan, the physician group, or the network generally begins with the completion of a form by a physician. This form typically asks the physician to complete information with respect to educational background, including schools and residencies attended and completed, and state licenses to practice medicine. In addition, information is elicited about whether the physician is board certified or eligible in any specialties and whether the physician participated in any additional educational activities and continuing professional medical education programs. Information about the nature and type of privileges which the physician has at hospitals may be sought, along with information concerning the revocation or suspension of such privileges. Information about malpractice lawsuits against the physician, any malpractice judgments or settlements, or conviction of any crimes also may be requested, and the National Practitioners Data Bank might be queried.

Additional information sought in the credentialing process includes the nature of the physician's professional liability insurance, its limits per occurrence and in the aggregate, and whether such insurance has ever been denied, suspended, canceled, or not renewed. In addition, whether the policy is an occurrence policy or claims made policy may be requested, along with assurance that tail insurance will be available and will be purchased. Further, the name of the insurer often will be requested, and sometimes a certificate of insurance, as well.

A health plan may request information about physicians' affiliations with medical groups; their practice locations; whether they have or have had any medical condition which might interfere with their ability to practice medicine, and whether they had been treated or advised to seek treatment for alcohol or other substance dependency. A physician who was ever employed in a setting where he or she was practicing medicine might be asked whether such employment was ever terminated by an employer. In addition, the physician might be asked whether his or her license to practice medicine, DEA registration or other narcotics license, hospital or other healthcare facility staff membership or privileges, professional organization membership, Medicare, Medicaid, state medical board or HMO, PPO, or prepaid health plan participation was denied, revoked, suspended, not renewed, placed under probation, curtailed, and so on.

Other information may be requested by the managed care plan in the credentialing process in order to determine whether the physician meets the standards for becoming a credentialed physician by the health plan. The credentialing process is important to ensure that quality physicians are providing healthcare services to a managed care plan's patients or enrollees. In addition, a managed care plan will want to ensure that it only has credentialed quality physicians, to minimize any risk it might have for not doing so.

Larger medical groups and integrated delivery systems also seek to credential their physicians. Such a process is new to many physicians who have practiced in small groups where all the physicians were partners and they decided to add physicians only as the need arose: they interviewed a prospective physician, spoke with colleagues about the physician's qualifications, and made a hiring decision. In the larger physician groups and integrated delivery systems, the physicians do not know each other, or their qualifications, as well, and it is necessary to ensure that physicians who become part of the group or integrated delivery system meet certain quality standards. It also is necessary to have this information readily available for the health plans. Much of the information elicited by medical groups is similar to that requested by the health plans.

COORDINATION OF THE CREDENTIALING PROCESS

The physician group or integrated delivery system likely will coordinate the credentialing process on behalf of its physicians for the managed care plans with which it contracts. As a result, current credentialing information will be kept by the group or the integrated delivery system on each physician. For example, whenever a physician renews his or her license or insurance coverage (unless it is acquired by the group or the integrated delivery systems on behalf of the physicians), or obtains additional continuing medical education credits, he or she should provide such documentation to the medical group or the system. When the managed care plans request additional information about physicians in the medical groups or systems, need updated information, or initially credential such physicians in the case of a new plan contracting with the group or the system, the information can be taken from the physician's updated files.

Increasingly, the burden of assembling such information by physicians for numerous health plans decreases the amount of time a physician has available to practice medicine. As a result, large groups or systems which can coordinate the collection of such information on behalf of the physicians can save physicians' time, thus affording them more time for patient care activities.

IMPORTANCE OF CREDENTIALING

Physician groups and networks have turned to the credentialing of physicians in the group or the network to ensure that only quality physicians are practicing in such groups and networks. Increasingly, however, such groups and networks are interested in ensuring that the physicians practicing with the group or network provide cost-effective treatment. Such a consideration is very important where the medical group or network is fully capitated or at risk for the services which it provides because it receives a fixed payment pmpm.

A health plan also will be concerned with a physician's ability to render cost-effective care, but as long as it has capitated a medical group or network its main concern will be whether the group or network is financially viable and whether it delivers quality care. A few, high-cost overutilizing physicians are the liability of the medical group or the network in such an arrangement. Their cost-ineffective provision of medical care can result in substantially higher costs for the group or the network, resulting in overcompensation to the physicians—in effect, the cost-effective physicians subsidize the less cost-effective physicians in the group, absent a physician compensation mechanism which takes into account these factors.

ECONOMIC CREDENTIALING

Although physician groups have vigorously opposed economic credentialing by hospitals in the privileging process, with the shift toward managed care and capitation, physicians are leading the way in developing economic credentialing to ensure that the physicians who practice in their groups and networks do so cost-effectively.

Such credentialing decisions should be made by the physicians in the medical group or network setting; they should not be within the purview of any medical staff of a hospital. Hospital credentialing and privileging processes should be kept separate from medical group and network credentialing.

In fact, although a network may conduct the ministerial aspects of physician credentialing, such as preparing information for the applications and review of same, the physicians should determine whether a physician will be credentialed as part of a medical group or a network. This is particularly important in networks which might be considered hospital-controlled or based because it is preferable that the hospital not be involved in this process. As managed care proliferates, and many physicians are closed out of such contracts by not being a part of medical groups or networks with managed care contracts, such excluded physicians will find it difficult to maintain a livelihood. As a result, it is likely that the frequency of lawsuits challenging exclusion from medical groups and networks will increase, as will decisions to remove physicians from medical groups and networks.

As a result, much care must be taken by physicians making credentialing decisions to ensure that they are based on criteria which will be upheld by the courts. Of course, a decision by three primary care physicians in a group to add a fourth physician can be based on just about whatever criteria the other three physicians want to employ. However, in a network of 200 physicians, the standards may be much more complicated, and physicians closed out of such networks, or terminated, may resort to the courts for redress. If the group or network is not truly integrated and is the only means of accessing health plans in an area, a physician may be able to fashion an argument that he or she should not have been excluded from a group or network.

It should be noted that it is much easier to exclude a physician from a medical group or network in the first instance than to terminate a physician from the group or the network once he or she becomes part of it. As a result, providers should be careful developing overly inclusive networks as a means to include all those physicians who desire to participate. Such overinclusion may lead to difficult decisions in the future with costly ramifications.

CONCLUSION

Managed care plans, physician groups, and networks generally perform some form of physician credentialing. Much information is sought about a physician's background in an attempt to ensure that the physician is a quality provider. The credentialing process can be coordinated on behalf of the physician to facilitate its completion. Finally, although physicians have opposed economic credentialing by hospitals, they are leading the way in economic credentialing in their groups and provider networks to ensure their economic viability in a competitive managed care environment.

12

Specialty Medical Groups, Networks, and Ancillary Providers—Alternatives to Fully Integrated Delivery Systems

With all the focus on primary care physicians and integrated delivery systems, one might wonder why more specialty medical groups are forming. Specialists who might have traditionally practiced in a solo or dual setting are often not courted by integrated delivery systems which focus on primary care. When they are sought, the view is held that they will have to contract at any rate and thus they can be brought into the system later.

Specialists are feeling the effects of the changing healthcare system, capitation, and the development of integrated delivery systems on their pocketbooks. They also see themselves being divided, lost, and relegated to an unimportant position in the new marketplace. They are concerned that quality has taken a back seat to price, and they see what little autonomy they have left in today's healthcare system eroding further.

SPECIALTY MEDICAL GROUPS

Some specialists have sought to create specialty medical groups which would help to preserve some specialty physician autonomy. Many of these groups hope that they can develop more effective practice parameters and treatment protocols because their groups will be focusing on the specialists and not the primary care physician. Integrated delivery systems, of course, focus on primary care physicians, and in doing so, when they begin to develop the practice parameters and protocols necessary in the efficient, cost-effective treatment of patients, they start initially with the PCPs. With the development of specialty medical groups, there can be an immediate focus on the particular specialty aspects of practice, resulting in greater efficiency for the physicians in the specialty medical group.

As noted above, it is particularly important for specialists planning to accept capitalization, to ensure that they have a significant and sufficient number of lives for which they are financially responsible. The development of a specialty medical group makes it possible for the specialty physician to be a more meaningful participant in any integrated delivery system, not merely a small part or division of a larger entity. As a result, if the specialty medical group can practice in a cost-effective manner and offer a low price to another physician group in an integrated delivery system, it might be more likely to contract with such a specialty medical group in lieu of contracting with or employing one or a limited number of specialists.

The primary care physician group or integrated delivery system contracting with the specialty group might not need to provide the specialty group with as many capitated lives to convince it to enter into a capitation arrangement, because the specialty group can aggregate enrollees for which it might be capitated by other primary care medical groups and integrated delivery systems. Thus, specialty medical groups which participate in more than one system may be able to capitate sooner and reduce their risk because they are likely to be responsible for a greater number of capitated patients.

CHARACTERISTICS OF SUCCESSFUL SPECIALTY MEDICAL GROUPS

There are certain characteristics of a successful, specialty medical group under capitation. These include ensuring that the specialty medical group has a sufficient number of lives under capitation to reduce its risk of providing medical services and a limited number of specialists to ensure that it has a sufficient number of lives per physician in the group.

The specialty group probably will want to practice in a broad geographic area with a diverse patient population, and at a number of facilities or sites to ensure that it will have a sufficient number of capitated lives to reduce its risk and to make its agreement economically beneficial to the specialists. In addition, it will want to be able to serve those lives in a manner consistent with the best interests of the patients. It also might be part of a larger IDS which has the necessary lives under contract for the specialty medical group.

Last, but not least, the specialty medical group needs to successfully manage care and recognize that primary care is the focus of a successful delivery system. Specialty physicians who combine in specialty physician groups in an attempt to preserve the practice of medicine in the form it was in 10 or 15 years ago will have a difficult time succeeding. Such groups are likely to tend toward decreasing, modified fee-for-service payments in lieu of capitation payments. The incentives will not be aligned in their system, with the result that their cost of providing services may not be managed as appropriately.

TYPES OF SPECIALTY MEDICAL GROUPS

Specialty medical groups may be single specialty or multispecialty in nature. A single specialty medical group focuses on one specialty. It may consist of anesthesiologists, oncologists, neurosurgeons, or any other single specialty group of physicians. The nature of the single specialty medical group will, of course, help determine its focus.

Anesthesiology groups often practice as hospital-based physicians, but also provide services at ambulatory surgery centers and possibly other settings. Such single specialty groups may be part of the package pricing of surgical services, a subcontractor to a medical group or integrated delivery system, or a direct contractor to a health plan.

An oncology group may combine physician and certain ancillary services in a global or package price, or seek to obtain a capitated amount from another physician group, such as a primary care group, or from a health plan.

A neurosurgery group likely will be willing to take capitation only if the group has a much greater number of lives than the oncology group to minimize the risk of capitation. Generally, it will want to contract on a modified fee-for-service basis. However, in the future many such groups might be paid according to APGs.

In addition to single specialty medical groups, many multispecialty medical groups are emerging. A multispecialty medical group may consist of physicians of two or more specialties, but it will likely consist of the major subspecialties most often required by patients. These groups can spread the capitation risks among many specialties. Multispecialty medical groups can even contract with primary care groups to provide all the specialty care for the primary care medical group. Such a contract can be a form of one-stop shopping for the primary care group; thus, the group avoids having to contract with numerous single specialty groups or individual physicians.

The primary care physicians ideally would capitate the multispecialty medical group for all the specialty and subspecialty services. The issue of individual specialty compensation would thus be left to the specialists.

SPECIALTY MEDICAL GROUP PARTICIPATION IN NETWORKS

As mentioned above, integrated delivery systems will seek to capitate all specialists over time. With the shift toward primary care based systems and medical groups, specialty and multispecialty medical groups can become owners in or contractors to such systems and medical groups. For example, a specialty medical group could be an owner in a PHO in addition to a separate physician organization. An example of this model is set forth in Figure 12-1.

In lieu of being an owner in the PHO, a specialty medical group might merely be a subcontractor to the physician organization. Although the specialists may not have an equity interest in the PHO, they may seek a long-term contractual relationship with the physician organization. Such a model, however, does not ensure continued access to the capitation revenues because the agreement between the specialists and the physician organization can be terminated. An example of the model where the specialty medical group is a subcontractor to the physician organization component of a PHO is set forth in Figure 12-2.

Even with a fully integrated delivery system consisting of one corporation with a hospital division and a physician practice division, the specialty medical group might be a subcontractor to the physician practice division. For example, the physician practice

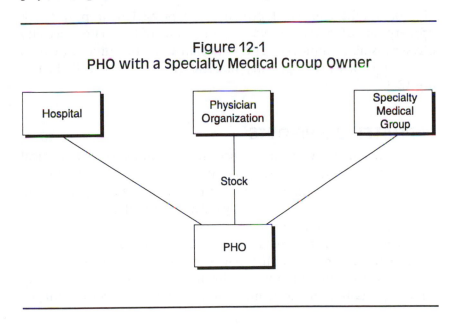

Figure 12-1
PHO with a Specialty Medical Group Owner

Figure 12-2
PHO with a Specialty Medical Group as a
Subcontractor to Physician Organization

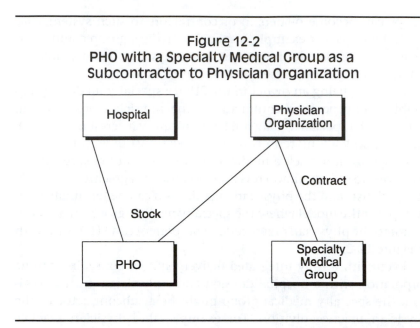

division might consist of primary care physician employees, or primary care physician employees with some of the major specialty physicians also employed. The physician's practice division would subcontract with the specialty medical group, as set forth in Figure 12-3.

CAPITATED CARVE-OUTS

The arrangements whereby a specialty or multispecialty medical group receives a subcapitated amount from a physician group or a capitated amount from a health plan is known as a capitated carve-out. Capitated carve-outs also may exist in a number of other areas One of the best examples is mental health.

For years, many managed care organizations and employers have realized that mental health services might be best managed and contracted for with employers or health plans through a company which specializes in the management of mental health managed

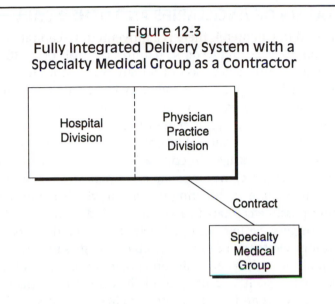

Figure 12-3
Fully Integrated Delivery System with a
Specialty Medical Group as a Contractor

care, such as Green Spring Health Services, Inc., of Maryland. Green Spring and companies like it charge a premium for a package of mental health benefits, and either contract with, employ, or purchase the provider portion of the system to ensure that they have adequate provider capacity. Through the development of practice parameters, protocols, and other means, mental healthcare is managed in a cost-effective manner.

Continual advances have been made in the last few years in the area of mental health treatment. More care has been moved to an outpatient basis, and partial hospitalization programs have become more prevalent. With a partial hospitalization program, the patient does not stay in the hospital 24 hours, but is treated and released during the day.

Other major capitated carve-out areas include vision and dental plans. These plans, while more likely to be an add-on in healthcare coverage, are increasingly seeking to capitate their providers for the services which they provide.

CAPITATION OF ANCILLARIES AND OTHER CARVE-OUTS

As discussed in Chapter 4, there is a movement to capitate laboratories and pharmacies, but to do so requires controls on utilization to ensure that the physicians do not merely order more tests or drugs because the laboratory or drug company is capitated. One means of assuring that the laboratory or pharmacy services will not be indiscriminately used by the physician ordering the tests or the pharmaceuticals is the use of financial incentives. For example, if the physician under- or overutilizes in comparison to the average physician with a similar practice, the physician's compensation may be reduced unless there is some extenuating reason for what the physician did.

Other possible capitated carve-outs include cancer centers, ambulatory surgery centers, and pediatric integrated delivery systems. An oncology center can capitate for all oncology services, including all hospital services; whereas an oncology group, unless it owns or contracts with such a center, is likely only to contract for the physician services and the associated ancillary services.

ASCs AS A SPECIAL CASE

Ambulatory Surgery Centers (ASCs) present an interesting case. In the 1980s, many freestanding ASCs did very well financially by controlling costs and ensuring that as many procedures as possible were performed in the center. In fact, many were established as joint ventures with a number of physicians who would be likely to refer patients to the freestanding ASC. If the ASC was more profitable, the referring physician investor might receive a dividend payment on a yearly or other basis as a profit distribution from the ASC.

Typically, the charges and costs of a hospital-based ASC far exceeded those of a freestanding ASC. With the development of integrated delivery systems led by hospitals and physicians, however, ASCs are finding it difficult to find their place because hospitals want to use their own surgical capacity. When the physicians of the IDS have their own ASC, they want to use it.

Ironically, efficient and economic use of ASCs might have been at the cornerstone of IDS development. With the greater movement to outpatient procedures, many of which are surgical in nature, and with ASCs operating more efficiently and economically than hospital surgery centers, ASCs should be playing an important role in integrated delivery systems and in keeping the costs of providing healthcare as low as possible on a pmpm basis.

There are, however, significant roadblocks to ASC participation in IDS. The most often encountered roadblock is the desire of the hospital to use its own outpatient surgical services. Although these services are often high in costs, the hospital looks at its variable cost of providing ASC services and often decides to use its own capacity. Part of the reasoning is that it is a cost of the system in any event.

Although another roadblock might be the physician ownership of a freestanding ASC, it may be a low-cost provider in any event; as a result, the physicians participating in the IDS may desire to sell their ASC to the IDS. However, the ASC could contract directly with the IDS, or if it has been contracting directly with the health plans, it may desire to continue to do so. It could contract directly with the health plans on a fee schedule or capitated basis, as a contractor through a medical group or through a hospital. Finally, as noted above, the ASC could be owned by the IDS.

PEDIATRIC CARVE-OUTS

There is a movement to carve pediatrics out of the general adult healthcare system and to create pediatric integrated delivery systems which contract with health plans on a capitated basis for all hospital and physician care rendered to children. Where health plans will not carve out pediatrics, pediatric medical groups or pediatric integrated delivery systems seek to subcontract through other adult-based medical groups and integrated delivery systems.

The development of pediatric integrated delivery systems is important in the preservation of quality healthcare for children. It is generally thought best for a child to receive care from a primary care pediatrician or a pediatric subspecialist because such a physician is trained in the special healthcare needs of children. Similarly, children's hospitals are thought best able to care for children. A pediatric integrated delivery system seeks to preserve the pediatric physician network and children's hospital care for children.

A preferred method of developing a pediatric integrated delivery system is to start with a primary care-based pediatric medical group which has experience appropriately managing care and then develop or build a specialty pediatric physician component. One means of developing that component is by contracting with a faculty practice plan. However, care must be taken to ensure that the high costs of the faculty practice are not charged to the primary care pediatricians or to the pediatric integrated delivery system. The special situation of academic medical centers and faculty practice physicians is discussed in Chapter 13.

The primary care pediatric medical group could be a division of a major children's hospital or a community hospital, or it could link by contract. The service area for the pediatricians likely will have to be large to ensure that there are enough capitated pediatric lives to ensure the success of the system, that is, enough to support the contracting or employed pediatric specialists and subspecialists. The number of lives necessary will far exceed those for an adult system.

One example of a developing pediatric integrated delivery system is the Northern California Pediatric Health System and its link with the Northern California Pediatric Medical Group, both based in Palo Alto, California. The Northern California Pediatric Medical Group is an IPA consisting of over 65 pediatricians serving the San Francisco Bay Area. The Northern California Pediatric Health System is an MSO owned and operated by the Lucile Salter Packard Children's Hospital at Stanford. The Medical Group contracts with the Pediatric Health System for managed care contract negotiations, information system needs, and other services. The physician specialty component of care is to be provided by a PHO consisting of the pediatric portion of the faculty practice program of the Stanford Health Services and by community and other subspecialists. The idea is that children should be the focus of the system and should not have to travel too far for specialty healthcare unless it cannot be provided in their community.

CONCLUSION

Specialty medical groups have been created to preserve some physician autonomy. Such groups seek to contract with primary care groups or directly with health plans on a capitated or other basis to provide specialty medical services to the group or health plan's patients. To be successful, such groups need to possess or develop the characteristics of a successful specialty medical group. There are myriad specialty medical groups, and there are a variety of ways that they can compete in networks.

Capitated carve-outs exist in a number of areas, such as mental health, vision, and dental, and are emerging in a number of areas, such as for laboratory and pharmaceutical services. Ambulatory surgical centers and pediatrics also create opportunities for carve-outs.

13

Academic Medical Centers

Academic medical centers present a special case in managed care and integrated delivery system development. Although they are typically seen as high-cost providers with faculty practice plans that likewise are high-cost, they can play a role in managed care and integrated delivery systems development.

Many academic medical centers had the foresight to envision the changing market, and affiliated with or developed alliances with community hospitals and other providers. As freestanding hospitals were looking for partners, those academic medical centers which were willing to enter into such affiliations and lend their name to those institutions were able to start to create healthcare systems. Those academic medical centers which developed or aligned with primary care physicians and developed physician networks positioned themselves to compete in the market of the 1990s; however, few appear to have been so forward thinking.

Most academic medical centers continued to train specialists in lieu of primary care physicians, were not interested in affiliating with community facilities which they viewed as inferior, and were not interested in developing a primary care component unless it was consistent with their academic mission. Most academic medical centers also were not interested in contracting with health plans on a capitated basis. Many believed that they rendered the top-quality services and that health plans would have to contract with them for certain tertiary and quaternary services in any event.

Certain academic medical centers may have been successful in securing contracts with managed care plans, but to a great extent those contracts were with PPOs or with HMOs where the HMO was assuring the availability of certain tertiary or quaternary services on a fee-for-service basis, not capitating the academic medical center and its physician components. Thus, the medical center does not control the lives, but merely provides services.

If the health plan assumes there are some services which it might need to purchase from an academic medical center, it is better if it contracts for all or part of those services at a discounted rate than paying billed charges. As a result, a health plan might always contract with academic medical centers for *certain* services. Academic medical centers often thought that health plans would have to contract with them for tertiary and quaternary care; however, many such centers have learned that they were not to be relied upon for all the tertiary and quaternary services that they thought they might provide. For example, many tertiary community hospitals provide cardiovascular and other specialty services, and have the contracts with health plans to do so. In fact, many have even developed outcomes analyses in the areas in which they provide tertiary and quaternary services, where those competing academic medical centers have not done so.

Of course, an academic medical center can contract on a modified fee-for-service basis with a health plan or integrated delivery system for the tertiary and quaternary services which it provides. However, in such a situation, the academic medical center is a true cost center, neither managing capitation payments (revenues) nor care. Some academic medical centers will face this plight. They will be subjected to continued cherry picking by health systems which likely will provide certain types of care if they can appropriately manage that care and it is profitable for them.

FOCUS OF ACADEMIC MEDICAL CENTERS

The focus of academic medical centers should be on developing relationships with community physicians, developing a primary care component through acquisition, or employment of physicians who can manage care. Where an academic medical center has its own employed or contracted physicians who have managed care, that division or organization will be the focus. The faculty specialty physicians can provide the specialty component.

COSTS OF ACADEMIC MEDICAL CENTERS

There is a common tendency to analyze the costs associated with an academic medical center, including the faculty practice plan, and to determine that the medical center and the plan is too costly in its provision of healthcare services. Before making that determination, however, academic medical centers and their faculty practice programs need to consider their true costs of providing services—for many, this is no simple task. To isolate such costs, academic medical centers and their faculty practice plans need to isolate their true costs of providing hospital and physician services and place the physicians in a responsible position for the costs which they can control.

In an academic environment, there are at least three cost components on the physician side, including the teaching function and the supervision of residents, the research component, and the cost of providing clinical services. It is often useful to determine what percentage of a physician's time is spent on each of these activities or the physician's estimate thereof. Next, the cost of providing those services and the revenues associated with them should be allocated. For example, if a faculty practice physician spends one-third of his or her time on the teaching function, and the academic medical center is paying the physician less for the teaching function than the physician's cost of providing such services including his or her salary, that difference should not be seen as an inefficiency in the physician provision of clinical services.

Often, internal costs, such as a dean's tax, are allocated to the physicians. Although it may be appropriate for the medical school to make whatever cost allocation it desires, it should be noted that such costs should not be allocated to the faculty practice plan to determine whether it is efficient in providing care.

After initially isolating the amount of time each member of the faculty practice plan spends providing clinical care, it is important to determine whether such physicians are actually providing care for that percentage of time and are available to do so. Occasionally, faculty practice physicians note that the allocation assigned to them for clinical care is not an allocation with which they agree and/or they have no intention of providing the necessary clinical care to fill the percentage to which they were assigned. The costs associated with such physicians should be adjusted to focus on the true costs of their actually providing clinical services on a full time equivalent basis. Once the true costs associated with the faculty practice plan's provision of care has been isolated, it is possible to determine the ability of the faculty to practice efficiently.

In addition, however, one must look at the nature of the patients which the faculty members are seeing. Often the very specialty nature of the physician practices results in the physicians being responsible for a very sick patient population. This factor must be figured into the equation.

On the hospital side, the true costs of the hospital should be determined, and prospective purchasers such as health plans should be made aware of the higher case mix of the academic medical center, and how that affects its cost structure.

THE DESIRE TO MANAGE CARE

Faculty practice physicians also must have the desire and the will to manage care to be successful in a managed care and integrated delivery system environment. Perhaps the liberal use of tests and procedures for research purposes should not be considered part of the cost of providing clinical care unless that is truly the means by which a physician provides clinical services for his or her patients.

Of course, if such is the case, certain faculty members will likely be the high-cost providers which they may be perceived to be.

The faculty must recognize that, in many academic settings, the ability of the physicians to continue to do much of the research they desire to do may depend on their ability to generate clinical practice revenues to subsidize such activities. Although academic medical centers and faculty practice physicians will continue to compete for grants, such competition is keen and not all research can be funded by grants. In addition, academic medical centers are finding it more and more difficult to pay physicians increasing amounts for their teaching functions. Faculty practice plans need to develop cohesive structures which strive to maximize their revenue from clinical practice to ensure that they remain viable entities, providing top-quality teaching, research, and clinical care.

In addition, the medical center itself should be committed to appropriate sizing and cost-effectiveness. It needs to recognize that it is a cost center.

ACADEMIC MEDICAL CENTERS AS LEADERS IN MANAGING CARE

Ironically, one might think that the faculty at academic medical centers would be less costly than other physicians. They are generally thought to be at the cutting edge of their practice areas. They should be in a position to implement practice parameters and protocols more quickly than their nonacademic counterparts because in many instances such physicians set the standard of care. In fact, in many such instances, it will be the faculty practice physicians who will set the standard of care in the community. Thus, the faculty practice physicians should be at the forefront of the technology curve, taking advantage of advancements in medical treatment and capitalizing on it.

The academic medical center should be working with the physicians to keep costs down through pursuing such developments. Of course, there are many areas where the high cost of technology may increase treatment costs, while saving a life or improving the quality of life. However, it is incumbent upon academic medical centers and faculty practice plans to be concerned not only with the aspect of providing cutting-edge medicine, but also with the cost of providing such services. As mentioned above, however, health plans should be educated as to the high case mix effect on the costs of the academic medical center.

PRACTICE AS USUAL

Of course, there may be academic medical centers with large endowments which will be in a financial position to accommodate practice as usual. However, it will be increasingly difficult for such medical centers to attract health plan contracts, even if the medical center is willing to lose money on such contracts. Health plans are looking for provider partners which can manage care. Those medical centers which can afford to practice as usual may survive—not because they were able to adapt to the marketplace of the mid-1990s, but because they had the endowments to subsidize their operations.

CONCLUSION

The most likely role for most academic medical centers in managed care will be one of the following two alternatives, which are not mutually exclusive: (1) anchors for fully integrated delivery systems, or (2) contractors to many delivery systems and health plans for the tertiary and quaternary care they provide. Those that have not set out on the first path years ago likely will find it difficult to do so now, and may be relegated to the second alternative.

14

Alliance, Contract, or Virtual Integration

Increasingly, physicians are recognizing that the high costs incurred by including hospitals as equity participants in integrated delivery systems may result in less monies available to the physicians. As a result, the physicians are seeking partners who have the capital of hospitals, but not the high costs associated with an asset-based system in the network. A likely partner for such physicians are health plans. Through alliance and contractual relationships, physicians are developing relationships which seek to replicate integrated delivery systems. These delivery systems which do not involve hospital ownership may be called alliance, contract, or virtual integration.

HEALTH PLANS AS PARTNERS FOR PHYSICIANS

Most health plans do not own hospitals or have high asset-based cost structures. Many have extensive capital, often exceeding that of the hospitals and the health systems. Health plans also have contracts with hospitals at discounted rates which they can make available for the benefit of the physician/health plan network. And most importantly, a health plan generally brings managed care lives to the physician/health plan relationship. In fact, the reason for the development of integrated delivery systems is to compete in the managed care arena, obtain managed care contracts, and be responsible for managed care lives. Health plan physician alliances help to accomplish these objectives.

In those states that allow it, the employment of physicians is an option for the health plan in developing such a network. In those states where a health plan can own an interest in a medical group, it may take an ownership interest in all or part of the physician group. The health plan also may contract with a medical group to provide services to the health plan's patients, either on an exclusive or nonexclusive basis.

THE HEALTH PLAN AS THE MSO

The health plan may act as a management services organization (either through a division or a subsidiary corporation) on behalf of the physicians, negotiating other managed care contracts on behalf of the physicians and possibly contracting directly with the hospitals for their services. The managed care plan and the physicians might prefer that other health plans contract directly with the health plan for the provision of all hospital and physician services, but understandably those other health plans will be reluctant to do so because they likely would not want to contract with a competitor. This built-in conflict will likely impede the development of such networks, but they will attempt to expand their base by management of network costs to enable the health plan to offer more attractive rates to employers.

Figure 14-1 is an example of a possible contract, alliance, or virtual integration model. In this model, the health plan creates an MSO division which provides services to a physician organization that contracts with the MSO to provide physician services for managed care patients. The physicians could be employed by the health plan, and the MSO division might provide the infrastructure for their practice. In addition to the health plan's contract with the physicians to provide services to the health plan's managed care patients, the MSO seeks to negotiate with other payors for managed care contracts

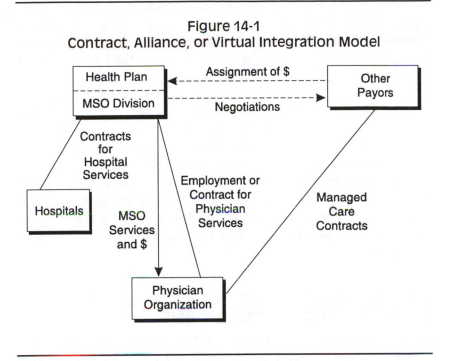

Figure 14-1
Contract, Alliance, or Virtual Integration Model

for the physician organization. The MSO division takes an assignment of such revenues, retains a fee for its services, and passes the remaining revenues to the physician organization. The health plan contracts with hospitals for hospital services and seeks to receive capitation payments for other health plans for the services the hospital provides, and pays it on a modified fee-for-service basis. For the health plan's patients, it merely pays the hospital on a modified fee-for-service basis, recognizing that it is a cost center.

TREATMENT OF THE HOSPITAL AS A COST CENTER

Such physician/health plan networks may be best able to manage care because they likely will be able to provide healthcare services at a lower cost than asset-based hospital networks. If such systems capture the hospital capitation payment for revenues which might have been available for hospital payments, the physicians—by controlling hospital admissions, lengths of stay, and the performance of procedures in the hospital—likely will be able to reduce the revenue to the hospital-contracting components of the system and increase the amount of revenues available to the physicians and the managed care plan. As a result, the health plan might even be able to decrease the cost of its premiums to employer groups. By stemming the increase in or decreasing such premiums, the health plan's products become more attractive to employer groups. If more attractive products lead to more employer groups contracting with the managed care plan, the physician/health plan network will be responsible for more managed care lives. It then can expand and become more successful.

EXPANSION OF CONTRACT, ALLIANCE, OR VIRTUAL INTEGRATION SYSTEMS

As noted above, health plan alliances and contractual relationships with physicians to develop a form of integrated delivery system without the ownership of hospitals is known as alliance, contract, or virtual integration. As alliance, contract, or virtual integration systems expand the number of lives for which they are responsible, they can begin to increase their asset base through cost-effective expansion. Such a system may purchase an ambulatory clinic, purchase or develop an ambulatory surgery center, purchase or develop a women's center, purchase or operate a skilled nursing facility or a home health agency. If it has a sufficient number of lives, it also might develop a short-stay hospital or purchase a community hospital at a low, financially viable price.

Physician/health plan integration systems should be careful, however, not to become asset based systems, with the result that they face the same cost problems as hospital based systems. They should be certain they have more than enough lives in their system for any provider asset which they develop or purchase, in lieu of contracting with such providers, or they face the prospect of losing one of their greatest assets—flexibility.

RESOURCE ALLOCATION AND MANAGEMENT OF CARE

Virtual integration systems are able to make resource allocation decisions and patient allocation decisions in a more cost-effective manner than hospital based systems. Hospitals have to improve and update existing plants and ensure state-of-the-art equipment and facilities to be competitive for hospital operations. Physician/health plan based systems merely can contract with those state-of-the-art systems.

These alliance or contract systems will steer patients to the lowest cost component of the system. For example, such a system likely will contract with the low-cost, freestanding, ambulatory surgical center in its geographic area for most ambulatory procedures, leaving to the hospital those ambulatory surgical procedures which cannot be performed at the freestanding facility or which, for quality of care concerns (perhaps because of fear of complications with the patient), should be performed at a hospital based facility.

The charges associated with a procedure at a freestanding ASC may be one-third those of a hospital based ASC. A hospital based integrated delivery system will undoubtedly desire to utilize its own facilities because they already represent a cost to the hospital. The virtual integrated delivery system will contract with the facility which offers the best price, provided it can ensure quality care.

A virtual integration model does not preclude the presence of a physician practice management company in the model. In fact, although many health plans have the expertise to manage care in the network, they do not have physician practice management expertise, which may be an important part of a virtual integration model. A health plan can develop such expertise internally by creating a physician practice operating division or subsidiary, or it may seek on behalf of the physicians and itself to align with such a physician practice management company.

SPECIAL CAUTION TO HOSPITALS

Hospitals developing integrated delivery systems must recognize that they face alliance, contract, or virtual integration models as competitors. As a result, they must ensure that they approach their integration efforts without a fixation on their costs and without an attempt to penalize the physicians for the costs of the hospital component.

CONCLUSION

Although contract, alliance, or virtual integration offers an interesting alternative in the management of care and integrated delivery system development, the competitive aspects of contracting with other health plans may make their development difficult. However, in certain market areas, such integration models might be most effective.

15

Replication of the Physician Equity Model to Align Incentives

Much has been written about the desirability of the physician equity model and its ability to align incentives and manage care. (The physician equity model is discussed in Chapter 8.) It is true that incentives are aligned in a physician equity model, and the management of care is facilitated. However, in most such models it has been difficult for the physicians to accumulate capital, and as a result many have sought to partner with hospital systems, managed care companies, and large, for-profit management companies to satisfy their need for capital.

Physician practice acquisitions are often a large part of the development of integrated delivery systems. Often, physicians would rather be paid in cash or in the stock of an entity traded on one of the national exchanges in lieu of the stock of another medical group, particularly when the stock of that medical group may be restricted in its transferability, its marketability is limited, and its value uncertain and subject to significant fluctuations.

As a result, increasingly, parties are seeking to replicate the elements of a physician equity model without its limitations on access to capital. A first step in doing so is to ensure that, if the hospital operations of a system are cost-effective, the physicians share in that savings. For legal reasons, the development of such a system may require that it receive the hospital and physician capitation payments into one, central entity; that the hospital corporation leases its hospital facilities to the physicians; or that the physicians have the ability to take the capitation payment on behalf of the hospital.

HOSPITAL AND PHYSICIAN PAYMENTS CONTROLLED BY ONE ENTITY

If the hospital and physician capitation payments are paid into one central entity in the system, *e.g.*, a health plan or entity which can assume risk in a given state, that entity may attempt to allocate the capitation payments in a manner that replicates the equity model. That is, it may treat the physicians as if they own the hospital. An example of such a situation would be to set a budget for hospital payments and to pay the hospital a fixed amount pmpm based on a certain number of hospital inpatient lives per thousand, *e.g.*, 160. If the physicians do not meet that target, and days per thousand exceed 160, the hospital might be entitled to more payments. If the physicians keep the days per thousand below 160, the physicians might share in the hospital revenue to a certain extent. The idea is that if the physicians would have owned the hospital and days per thousand were up, they would make less money. If they kept days per thousand down, they would have made more money. The budgeted amount accounts for the fact that the physicians do not have control over all the hospital operations.

LEASE OF HOSPITAL FACILITIES

In a for-profit system, the hospital owners might lease the hospital to the physicians for a fixed payment, thus permitting the physicians the ability to have the hospital under their control aligning incentives. The entity which owns the hospital can perform other network functions for which it may receive network revenues. In fact, such a model reduces the hospital entity's desire to ensure that the hospital services are used. If the hospital entity is receiving a lease payment, it should be covering its fixed costs of owning the hospital.

HOSPITAL AND PHYSICIAN PAYMENTS PAID TO PHYSICIANS

If a physician group can be paid by the health plan for both the hospital and physician services component, it should be possible to replicate the equity model because the physicians can purchase the hospital services.

If the physicians, however, want to ensure access to the hospital's capital, and they are able to take the capitation payments on behalf of the hospital, they can treat the hospital as a cost center, but they also will need to treat the hospital as a partner. The hospital should demonstrate how it can add value to such a system. An important consideration will be whether the physicians can participate in the monies saved by the control of hospital costs. It is likely that to do so an arrangement will have to be developed to minimize the legal risks of this alternative. If the physicians can take both the hospital and physician capitation payments, or a health plan that is affiliated with the physicians does so, the legal risks may be minimized.

CONCLUSION

Is the physician equity model or replication of such model the only successful model for a fully integrated delivery system? The answer is an unqualified no. Many nonprofit integrated delivery systems exist which do a superb job of managing care and operate in a fully integrated manner. The Henry Ford Health System in Detroit, Michigan, is an example of such a system.

The physician equity model and its replication are only examples of models that might work in specific instances. This chapter only suggests a few alternatives. Many more can be developed. Each area of the country is different—its penetration of managed care, its compliment of physicians and hospitals, and its attractiveness to for-profit management companies. The management of care and the development of an integrated delivery system to manage care is a concept which must be embraced by the parties as a desirable goal. The form of such organization might be as varied as a diamond. A larger size will not necessarily result in a better system. The composition of the network and its ability to manage care will make the difference. If replication of the physician equity model helps facilitate the development of a network to manage care effectively and compete in a capitated environment, such an alternative should be considered.

16

Miscellaneous Legal Issues in Managed Care

Many laws affect the management of care and the development and operation of managed care companies, and integrated delivery systems. Many of these laws have been mentioned briefly earlier in this book. This chapter merely highlights a number of the major legal issues affecting managed care and integrated delivery systems. It does not address all such legal issues, and its treatment is by no means exhaustive or a substitute for competent legal advice. Managed care and integrated delivery system development and operations present many complicated legal issues which call for the assistance of competent counsel.

LICENSING/CERTIFICATION/REGULATION

As noted in Chapter 11, states regulate the practice of insurance, specifically the assumption of risk by a company to provide needed healthcare services to a defined patient population for a set price. HMOs, healthcare service plans, and indemnity carriers assume such risks. Although indemnity carriers are often state-regulated insurance carriers, healthcare service plans and HMOs are often governed by other laws which may be within the purview of a State Department of Insurance or Corporations. Healthcare service plans, such as the

Blue Cross and Blue Shield Plans, often have been regulated by separate statutes, and the special nature of HMOs generally results in a separate statutory scheme for these entities. PPOs may or may not be regulated by a state. Those that act only on behalf of other entities and assume no risk are less likely to be subject to regulation. There is a movement in some states to license and regulate PHOs and MSOs which seek to take risk.

States may require the licensing and/or certification of managed care entities. To become licensed or certified, the managed care entity must meet certain state requirements which are likely to include certain tests of financial solvency, reserves, assurances of adequate provider networks, and ability to arrange necessary service for their patient population. An HMO can become federally qualified, and to do so, it will have to meet requirements set by the regulatory and licensing schemes. Where a PHO or MSO takes capitated risk, a state may require that it be licensed in some form. More fully integrated delivery systems may face licensing and regulatory considerations, but they likely will be applied to the individual entities which comprise the IDS.

LAWS REGULATING TAKING RISK

State laws often regulate what entities can take risk for hospital and physician services. If the PHO or MSO seeks to take risk, it may, like an HMO, need to meet certain state requirements for solvency and financial reserves. In addition, it may be subject to the types of licensing, certification, or regulatory issues mentioned above.

Physicians and hospitals which seek to take risk or capitated payments for services they do not provide may encounter similar regulatory hurdles. There also may be an interplay with the prohibition against the corporate practice of medicine and medical practices acts which exist in some states. That is, if a PHO, MSO, or hospital cannot provide physician services, it may not be able to contract for the provision of such services and assume risk, absent a contrary position by the state department of insurance or corporations.

ANY WILLING PROVIDER LAWS

To be successful, managed care anticipates that networks will be restrictive in nature. As a result, managed care plans negotiate contractual arrangements for discounts with providers because providers expect that the network will be limited in scope and the physician or hospital likely will receive a substantial amount of business from the health plan.

Some states have enacted, or are attempting to enact, any willing provider laws which seek to require health plans to permit any provider willing to provide services to the health plan's patients at a certain price the ability to do so. Such laws are sometimes known as anti–managed care laws, as they undermine the underlying tenet of a successful managed care arrangement—they seek to expand the provider network, in lieu of restricting it; they adversely affect the management of care.

LAWS RESTRICTING UNDERUTILIZATION

In a capitated managed care situation, it is important to ensure that the providers render quality care and do not underutilize services. As a result, state laws often prohibit providers from denying services or withholding treatment to patients because of their status as managed care patients, and individuals or entities from paying such providers anything of value as an inducement to do so. In addition, federal law prohibits HMOs contracting under Medicare and Medicaid from failing "substantially to provide an enrollee with required medically necessary items and services and the failure adversely affects or has the likelihood of adversely affecting the enrollee. . . ."[5]

However, it should be noted that the very nature of managed care is the providing of cost-effective quality care, which involves the minimization of the costs of providing healthcare services to a defined patient population. In attempting to do so, the quality of those services must always be at the forefront to ensure proper compliance with these laws.

LAWS PROHIBITING PROVIDERS FROM BILLING OR SURCHARGING HMO PATIENTS

When a provider enters into a contractual arrangement with an HMO to provide services to its patient population, the provider must agree not to charge the patient or beneficiary for any services, except for applicable deductibles, if any, copayments, and noncovered services for which the patient has agreed in writing to pay prior to the delivery of those services. Applicable state and federal laws prohibit the provider from billing the beneficiary in such situations.

WAIVER OF DEDUCTIBLE AND COPAYMENT AMOUNTS

Many managed care plans take the position that if a provider waives a deductible or coinsurance amount, it is in violation of its contract with the managed care plan and in violation of applicable state laws. The health plan wants to be certain that the provider charges and collects the applicable copayment and deductible amounts to ensure that the incentives it has built into the system are adhered to by the provider and are working to accomplish the desired objectives. For example, if the health plan believes that a ten-dollar ($10) copayment will minimize excessive visits to the primary care physician, it would not want those copayments waived. State laws may govern the waiver of deductibles and coinsurance indirectly through interpretation of the state insurance laws. Where the provider is not being paid on a capitated basis but is being paid in part based upon its charges, the waiver of a deductible or copayment may be interpreted as the provider reducing its charge for services to the patient without providing the benefit of same to the health plan.

For example, if the health plan pays a provider based on 80% of its charges, and the applicable copayment is 20%, for $100 in charges the health plan should pay the provider $80 and the copayment should be $20. If, however, the provider waives the copayment of $20, the plan may contend that the provider's charge was really $80 and it should only pay 80% of that amount, or $64. In addition, as noted above, applicable state insurance law may support the plan's charge to the provider of a violation of those laws for representing that the provider's charge is higher than it was.

ANTITRUST LAWS

The antitrust laws govern the ability of managed care companies and providers to merge, acquire additional companies, and consolidate. They also govern network development and other aspects of managed care. On September 27, 1994, the U.S. Department of Justice and the Federal Trade Commission (the "Agencies") issued Statements of Enforcement Policy and Analytical Principles Relating to Health Care and Antitrust. These statements should be consulted in analyzing the antitrust aspects of managed care and integrated delivery systems.

As noted in Chapter 7, whether a physician group has achieved true integration of its assets and liabilities and is an integrated medical group or whether it accepts capitation payments will affect the antitrust scrutiny of its contracting arrangements. An integrated medical group can make joint decisions on managed care contracts and pricing. An IPA or CWW which is not integrated may be able to jointly negotiate managed care contracts if the payment under those contracts is on a capitated basis because there is enough sharing of risk in that situation, as each physician is financially responsible for the care rendered to that enrollee. With contracting on a modified fee-for-service basis, such as PPO contracting, a messenger should be employed to present the contract rate to the providers in the non-integrated group, and they should accept or reject those contracts on an individual basis, unless there is some substantial withhold. If the group withholds a substantial part of the fee-for-service revenue, and pays it back to the providers based on some minimization of cost formula while maintaining quality care, it may be possible for an IPA to contract with a health plan on such basis without running afoul of the antitrust laws. To be on the safe side, however, a nonintegrated group might want to apply to the Agencies for a business review letter approving of such an arrangement.

Although the antitrust laws do not permit the sharing of price information by competing providers, one of the new antitrust safety zones permits the sharing of information or data which could lead to the development of better treatment modalities, practice parameters, protocols, or clinical pathways.

With respect to the application of the antitrust laws to integrated delivery systems and their development, each aspect of the delivery system development should be analyzed under the antitrust laws. For example, the acquisition of another provider, the development of an exclusive arrangement with providers, and the nature of joint contracting decisions should be analyzed separately. The less exclusive in nature a system is, the less antitrust scrutiny there will be. Even if a network states that it is nonexclusive, but a number of considerations lead to the practical conclusion that the network is exclusive, it will be viewed by the government as an exclusive network. An example of an external factor which might lead to the conclusion that a network is exclusive is managed care plans that require that providers can contract only with the plan through one group or network. If such is the case with almost all health plans in an area, an integrated delivery system which does not require exclusivity of its physicians might be viewed by the Agencies as being exclusive.

The antitrust safety zones suggest that the physicians in an exclusive network should not exceed 20% of the physicians in the applicable market, and the physicians in a nonexclusive network should not exceed 30% of the physicians in the applicable market. In addition, the safety zone addresses the number and/or percentage of specialty physicians allowed in the network when there are a limited number of specialists in an area.

The Agencies have approved the development of purchasing cooperatives where large employer groups combine to negotiate lower rates with managed care plans. These purchasing cooperatives can have considerable market clout because of their size and the desire of the health plans to ensure that they retain or obtain the business of the employers in the cooperative.

The antitrust considerations in managed care and integrated delivery systems are too numerous to discuss fully in this chapter, but are important and should be carefully considered.

MEDICARE AND MEDICAID FRAUD AND ABUSE LAWS

The Medicare fraud and abuse laws prohibit payment for the referral of Medicare and Medicaid patients (the "antikickback laws"),[6] false claims to the Medicare or Medicaid program,[7] and myriad other relationships and transactions. For example, they also prohibit payment as an inducement to underutilize services,[8] violations of the Medicare "incident to" rules,[9] and the assignment of benefits.[10] The laws provide for possible criminal and civil penalties, the latter including substantial fines and possible exclusion from the Medicare and Medicaid programs. These laws exist on both the federal and state levels. There are safe harbors to the antikickback laws,[11] and they should be consulted with respect to certain managed care and integrated delivery system development, operations, and transactions.

The nature of a managed care plan's relationship with its providers is such that the plan seeks a discount from its providers because it is referring patients to those providers. There are safe harbors to the Medicare and Medicaid fraud and abuse laws which address managed care arrangements. One safe harbor addresses price reductions offered to health plans.[12]

As noted in Chapters 7 and 8, IDS development and operations are greatly affected by the Medicare fraud and abuse laws. There is no safe harbor for integrated delivery systems; rather, all aspects of the IDS development and its contractual relationships must be analyzed under the Medicare and Medicaid fraud and abuse laws. Such analysis begins with the acquisition of components of the IDS, *e.g.*, the acquisition of a physician group by a hospital. In such a situation, the government will want to ensure that as part of the purchase price for the medical group, no monies have been paid for the referral of patients to the hospital. Of course, if a managed care plan acquires a physician group, such concerns should not exist if neither party owns a hospital to which the physicians will be referring Medicare and Medicaid patients.

Any contractual relationships with the physicians should be analyzed to ensure there are no payments for the referral of patients.

That is, the physicians should be charged fair value for the services which they receive. In addition, their compensation should not exceed fair value. Ideally, the IDS would want to ensuré that the relationship met any Medicare safe harbor applicable to such arrangements.

STARK II SELF-REFERRAL AND STATE LAW PROGENY

The Ethics in Patient Referrals law, known as the Stark II self-referral law,[13] prohibits billing the Medicare and Medicaid programs for certain, designated services where the provider has an ownership or financial interest in the entity which provides such service. The objective of the law is to control overutilization of services from which a physician can benefit because of his or her ownership or financial interest in the entity.

The designated services to which the Stark law applies included, as of January 1, 1995:

- clinical laboratory services
- physical therapy services
- occupational therapy services
- radiology services
- radiation therapy services
- durable medical equipment
- parental and enteral nutrients, equipment, and supplies
- prosthetics, orthotics, and prosthetic devices
- home health services
- outpatient prescription drugs
- inpatient and outpatient hospital services

There are certain exceptions or arrangements which are excluded from the application of Stark II. These include, among others, the provision of services by certain truly integrated group practices, the provision of "in-office ancillary services," contracts for the rental of office space and equipment, *bona fide* employment relationships, and personal services arrangements. There are no blanket exceptions for managed care and integrated delivery systems. As with the Medicare fraud and abuse laws, the development of any entity or arrangement, and its operations and transactions, must be reviewed separately.

It should be noted that the physician self-referral prohibitions apply in a managed care arrangement to the extent that a physician refers a patient to a managed care organization, including a subsidiary provider or network, if the physician has a direct or indirect financial relationship with the organization, subsidiary provider, or network unless one of the exceptions is met. These include a prepaid plan exception which includes *certain* types of health plan organizations, the personal services arrangement exception, the employee exception, and the physician incentive plan exception. This latter exception may be met in part if "No specific payment is made directly or indirectly under the plan to a physician or a physician group as an inducement to reduce or limit medically necessary services provided with respect to a specific individual enrolled with the entity."[14]

Many states have enacted their own form of Stark self-referral laws. Some are broader, some are more restrictive, and some reference the federal law. These laws should be consulted on a state-by-state basis.

TAX EXEMPTION

It should be noted that although some health plans which seek IRS § 501(c)(3) status may be granted that status by the Internal Revenue Service if they independently qualify for such status, others only will obtain IRS § 501(c)(4) status. In the *Geisinger Health Plan* decision,[15] for example, it was noted that Geisinger did not qualify as a charitable organization under IRC § 501(C)(3) as an integral part of the Geisinger System, a related healthcare system exempt from taxation under IRC § 501(C)(3).

In integrated delivery system development, each entity must be reviewed by the IRS to determine whether it complies with the standards necessary to receive its tax exemption, and what form of exemption it receives. In addition, one must be careful with fully integrated, single corporation IDS to ensure that the operations of any one division do not raise unrelated business income issues or run afoul of certain state laws.

Relationships between the nonprofit entities in an integrated delivery system and the physicians or other insiders should be closely analyzed to determine whether there is any improper inurement of benefit or private benefit which might jeopardize the tax-exempt status of one or all of the nonprofit entities. Any contractual relationships with the physicians may be scrutinized to ensure that the physicians are paying fair value for the services which they receive and that any compensation to them is at fair value.

CONCLUSION

There are myriad laws and regulations which affect managed care and integrated delivery systems. This chapter only highlights a few of the major ones. Providers and health plans should ensure that they consult competent counsel to ensure they comply with applicable laws and regulations to the greatest extent possible, with a minimum of legal risk.

Endnotes

1. Glossary, Participants Manual, Pierce County Medical Bureau, Inc. (July 1992).

2. Glossary, Participants Manual, Pierce County Medical Bureau, Inc. (July 1992).

3. 42 C.F.R. § 410.26 and Part B Carrier's Manual (HIM- 14) § 2050.1.

4. 42 C.F.R. § 424.73(b)(3).

5. 42 C.F.R. § 1003.103(f)(1)(i) (1994).

6. 42 U.S.C. § 1320a–7b(b).

7. 42 U.S.C. § 1320a–7b(a).

8. 42 U.S.C. § 1320a–7a(b)(1).

9. See note 3.

10. See note 4.

11. 42 C.F.R. § 1001.952.

12. 42 C.F.R. § 1001.952(m).

13. 42 U.S.C. § 1395nn.

14. 42 U.S.C. § 1395nn(e)(3)(B).

15. *Geisinger Health Plan v. Comm'r of Internal Revenue*, Case No. 93–7699 (3rd Cir.) (July 28, 1994).

Index

Integrated medical group, 89
IPA model HMO, 16

J–K–L
Joint Commission on Accreditation of Healthcare Organizations (JCAHO), 52
Joint venture hospital and physician-owned MSO, 100, 102

Kaiser Permanent Health Plan, 2

Laboratories, capitation of, 11, 33, 43-44, 146
Legal issues, in managed care, 167-76
    antitrust laws, 171-72
    any willing provider laws, 169
    billing or surcharging HMO patients prohibited, 170
    licensing/certification regulation, 167-68
    medical foundations, 110
    Medicare/Medicaid fraud and abuse laws, 96, 173-74
    regulation of risk, 168
    restriction of underutilization, 169
    Stark II self-referral and state law progeny, 96, 174-75
    tax exemption, 175-76
    waiver of deductible and copayment amounts, 170-71
Liability insurance (physician), 134
Licensing regulation, 167-68
Lucile Salter Packard Children's Hospital, 148

M
Malpractice lawsuits, 133-34
Managed care contracts

see also Managed care organization(s)
    access to records, 66-67
    assignment of, 64-65
    appeals mechanisms, 62
    billing the beneficiary, 66
    boilerplate provisions, 70-71
    Catholic clause,70
    compensation, 53-55
    concurrent review, 57
    confidientiality, 69
    coordination of benefits, 68-69
    cost of record retrieval, audit, and photocopies, 67
    definitions, 50-52
    dispute resolution, 62-63
    exclusivity and incentives, 69
    grievance procedures, 63
    importance of, 78
    indemnity and/or hold harmless, 61-62
    independent contractors, 61
    insolvency of payor, 63-64
    insurance, 60-61
    most-favored nations clauses, 69-70
    nondiscrimination, 70
    parties to contract, 49-50
    prior authorization, 56-57
    proprietary rights and advertising, 65
    qualifications of provider, 52
    retrospective review, 57-58
    risk pools, 58
    services to be provided, 52-53
    term, 59
    termination of contract, 59-60
    utilization review/management and quality assurance, 55-56
Managed care organization(s), 14, 101

see also Managing care
-controlled integrated delivery system, 115, 117
integrated delivery systems and, 85-86
legal issues and, 167-76
-owned MSO, 101, 103
physician credentialing, 133-34
Management and quality assurance plans, 55-56
Management information systems, 129-30
Management services agreement, 98
Management services organizations, 13, 77-78, 93-102, 103
health plan as, 158-59
hospital-owned, 99, 100
independent corporations, 98
joint-venture hospital and physician-owned, 100, 102
managed care organization-owned, 101, 103
Medicare fraud and abuse laws, 99
outpatient centers and, 95
physician-owned, 99-100, 101
Managing care, 127-32
clinical or critical pathways, 128-29
commitment to, 130
management information systems, 129-30
outcomes analysis, 129
practice parameters, 127-28
protocols, 128
sufficient capitated population for, 131-32
workable model, 132
Market approach valuation, 107
Medicaid, 3
Ethics in Patient Referrals law and, 174

fraud and abuse laws, 173-74
risk plans, 22
termination of health plan contract, 60
Medi-Cal contracting, 5
Medical centers, academic, 151-56
costs of, 153-54
focus of, 153
as leaders in managing care, 155-56
Medical emergency, defined, 51
Medical foundations, 77-78, 106-10
hospital-owned or controlled, 108
tax-exempt status of, 107
with hospital division, 108, 109
without hospital division, 108-10
Medical group(s), 134
acquisitions, mergers, and consolidation of, 77
as basis for IDS, 90
development, and integrated delivery systems, 86-90
expansion, 75-77
importance of credentialing, 136
integrated, 89
Medical necessity, defined, 50-51
Medicare, 2-3, 4, 52
ambulatory payment groups and, 30
antikickback laws, 34, 95, 173
Ethics in Patient Referrals law and, 174
fraud and abuse, 79, 84, 89, 95, 99, 173-74
"incident to" rules, 94, 173
Resource Based Relative Value Scale payment schedule, 31
risk plans, 22
termination of health care contract, 60

About the Author

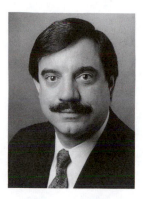

Paul R. DeMuro is a Partner in the Health Care Practice Group of the international law firm of Latham & Watkins, where he practices in the San Francisco and Los Angeles, California offices. He received his B.A. *summa cum laude* in Economics, from the University of Maryland, College Park; his M.B.A. in Finance from the University of California, Berkeley; and his J.D. from the Washington University, St. Louis. He is a CPA and a fellow in the Healthcare Financial Management Association (HFMA). He served on its National Principles & Practices Board from 1992 to 1995, and was Vice Chair from 1993 to 1995. His term on HFMA's National Board of Directors is from 1995 to 1997. He is a nationally recognized authority on managed care and integrated delivery systems and he has authored numerous publications and lectured extensively throughout the United States on such topics, and other health care subjects such as finance, Medicare reimbursement and fraud and abuse, antitrust, mergers and acquisitions, and nonprofit taxation. Mr. DeMuro is listed in *Who's Who in American Law* and the *Best Lawyers in America*. He lives in San Francisco with his wife and daughter.